MW00856916

DOCTOR-PATIENT HANDBOOK

by Bernard Jensen, D.C., Ph.D.

Dealing with the REVERSAL PROCESS
and THE HEALING CRISIS
through
Eliminating Diets and Detoxification.

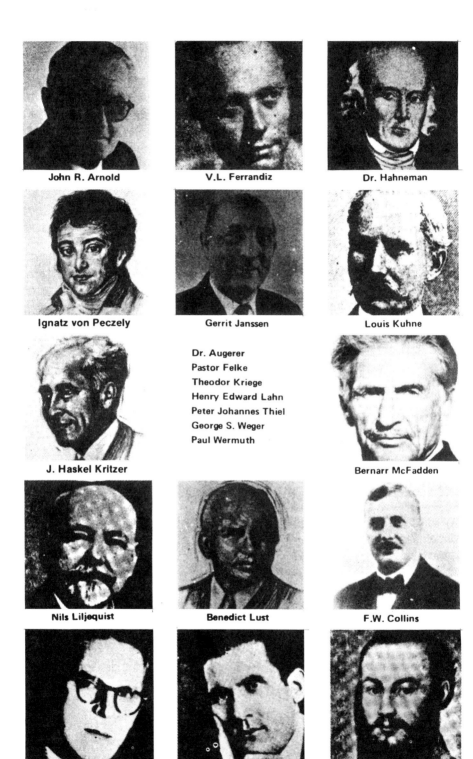

John R. Arnold

V.L. Ferrandiz

Dr. Hahneman

Ignatz von Peczely

Gerrit Janssen

Louis Kuhne

Dr. Augerer
Pastor Felke
Theodor Kriege
Henry Edward Lahn
Peter Johannes Thiel
George S. Weger
Paul Wermuth

J. Haskel Kritzer

Bernarr McFadden

Nils Liljequist

Benedict Lust

F.W. Collins

R.M. McLain

Marko J. Petinak

Ignatz von Peczely

Published by
Bernard Jensen International
24360 Old Wagon Road
Escondido, California 92027
Phone (619) 749-2727

Bernard Jensen, D.C., Ph.D.
Editor

"At thirty, man suspects himself a fool, Knows it at forty, and reforms his plan; At fifty, chides his infamous delay. Pushes his prudent purpose to resolve, In all the magnanimity of thought; Resolves, and re-resolves, then dies the same. And why? because he thinks himself immortal, All men think all men mortal but themselves."

—Young: Night Thoughts.

A Doctor-Patient Handbook discusses Elimination Diets and Detoxification with emphasis on the Reversal Process for Counteracting Chronic Diseases and The Healing Crisis.

On the cover are to be found photographs of doctors who strongly advocated natural treatment which brought on the Reversal Process and The Healing Crisis. All of these men worked with the Reversal Process in getting a person well by teaching good health, stopping the old way of living, taking on the new that built new tissue in its place. A brief summary of each doctor's contribution and specialty follows on the next pages.

DR. BERNARD JENSEN, D.C., N.D., Nutritionist, says it must be realized that what he has done in nature cure work is to follow the methods of the men who are presented in this book and with whom he studied. He has tried to carry on the precepts and activities of these men ... champions and geniuses in the healing art ... particularly in nature cure. They believed in it, they were dedicated to it, and they did a great amount of good for humanity by teaching people to live properly and follow the Nature Cure Way.

The Doctor-Patient Handbook

dealing with
The Reversal Process and The Healing Crisis
through
Elimination Diets and Detoxification

An Introduction to the Healing Approach and Philosophy
of
BERNARD JENSEN, D.C., Ph.D.

SUMMARY OF DOCTORS

DR. AUGERER of Germany — *Manual of Eye Diagnosis,* May 1953.

JOHN R. ARNOLD, D.C., born in Chicago, Illinois on July 30, 1896. Received his degree in 1925. Established World Iridology Fellowship and its Journal in June 1953. Has conducted numerous classes in Iridology for students and practitioners.

F.W. COLLINS — *Disease Diagnosed by Observation of the Eye,* 1908-19, Copyright 1919.

PASTOR FELKE lived from 1856 to 1926 in Germany. He was the first to realize, and indeed state openly, how infinitely valuable is especially the constitution diagnosis from the iris. He condensed the best in Naturopathy into a comprehensive therapeutic method — cold hip bath (modified according to Kuhne); air (breathing and moving exercises and air baths); light (action of light stimulation on the uncovered skin); earth (in the form of mud packs for sediment dissolving, draining, readjusting and defensive power). He valued the meatless diet and spoke up for use of raw food.

V.L. FERRANDIZ of Barcelona, Spain — *Iridiagnosis* (Spanish) 50 Chapters, 1st Edition 1970 — 810 pages, 6½x9½'', extensively illustrated in color (499 items). Iridology presentation is accompanied by related diagnostic procedures and subjects, pointing out interrelationship and manner in which Iridology plays such an important part in providing keys to answer questions, problems and differential considerations.

DR. HAHNEMAN — the Father of Homeopathy.

CONSTANTINE HERING — a Homeopath, gave us the Law of Cure showing that all cure is from within out. This law was worked out over many years through the process of elimination — how the body reversed over the tract in which it was developed.

GERRITT JANSSEN, Chiropractor, Herbalist and Naturopath since 1934. Born in Holland and spent ten years in the Far East. Resident of Australia beginning 1973. Pioneered much of Nature Cure work in Australia and has treated thousands of patients in that country. Vice President of the Australian Naturopathic Physicians Assn. and President of South Pacific Federation Natural Therapeutists, organized in 1967. Director of Triad Research Corporation developing iris photographic and analysis system. Strong advocate among farmers for organic farming methods.

BERNARD JENSEN, D.C., N.D., Nutritionist, of Los Angeles, California. Born in Stockton, Calif. in 1908. Graduated from West Coast Chiropractic College in Oakland, Calif., 1929. Studied with Dr. Benedict Lust and worked at his sanitarium in Butler, New Jersey, and spent a great deal of time in all types of post-graduate work, becoming well acquainted with the teachings of Dr. Tilden and Dr. Kellogg of Battle Creek fame. He holds many certificates of scholastic attainment from various schools and institutions. He became interested originally in Iridology by seeing Dr. J. Haskel Kritzer's book in the bookcase of his father, Dr. Eugen Jensen of Stockton. At the behest of Dr. R. M. McLain of Oakland, Calif., he began an intensive study and investigation of Iridology. Dr. McLain was the first man able to demonstrate to Dr. Jensen that Iridology was factual and workable. He completed course through the International School of Professional Arts and Science of Iridology with Dr. McLain as his teacher. Also, did four years of two nights a week of constant application of Iridology with patients under Dr. McLain's guidance. He drew 500 eyes in color before graduating from the American School of Naturopathy under guidance of Dr. F. W. Collins. Dr. Jensen has traveled and lectured extensively on Iridology in the U.S. and has also traveled in many foreign countries investigating the findings of Iridologists of those countries and accumulating devices used by them. His first lecture on Iridology was delivered at the convention of the American Naturopathic Association in 1931 at Milwaukee. During that same year he also taught Iridology at Dr. F. W. Collins' College in New Jersey and Dr. Benedict Lust's College in New York. The urge to "write a book" struck about 40 years ago and finally resulted in *The Science and Practice of Iridology*, Copyright 1952 USA and all countries signatory to Berne Convention. 2nd printing 1964, 3rd printing 1970, 4th printing 1973, 5th and copyright 1974.

JOHN HARVEY KELLOGG, M.D., who established the Battle Creek Sanitarium and the Battle Creek Health Methods. His work has stood as a monument to those who want to take care of their body in a good healthy way. He was a great believer in Ellen G. White, who wrote "The Ministry of Healing," and combined a wonderful outlook with his healing through natural methods. His great basic concept was changing the intestinal flora and taking care of the bowel. In this he was a Master. It is with him that I learned my first methods in the care of the bowel.

FATHER SEBASTIAN KNEIPP — Born May 21, 1821 in Bavaria. At the age of 26 he was given up to die with tuberculosis and through the spiritual thought in studying for his priesthood, he found, ''Go forth and touch thyself in the Jordan and thy flesh will again become healthy and clean.'' He became a great priest-healer using herbs and the water cure. His most wonderful volume is found in all natural cure libraries called *My Water Cure.* I spent much time in Worishofen, Germany where this water cure is practiced extensively. Father Kneipp was a master of The Water Cure, using cold water. He believed that cold water is live water and hot water is dead water. He treated as many as 4,000 people a week! He treated them with water and herbs. Camomile tea was an outstanding tea that he used for practically every patient.

THEODOR KRIEGE of Germany. Wrote a number of books on Iridology, his latest being *Foundation of Iridology* (German) and also available in English, released about February 1963.

J. HASKEL KRITZER, M.D., Los Angeles, California. *Textbook of Iridiagnosis and Guide to Treatment.* First Edition 1921, 7th Edition 1948. This Medical Doctor changed his methods of practice after seeing what Nature Cure could do.

LOUISE KUHNE of Leipzig, Germany — A discoverer in many ways of using the water cure methods in the pioneer stages of Nature Cure. Dr. Kuhne found the extreme values of building up the circulation of the bloodstream.

HENRY EDWARD LAHN [LANE], M.D., Chicago Illinois. *Iridology — The Diagnosis From the Eye,* entered at Library of Congress, Washington, D.C. and Stationers' Hall, London, 1904, 6th Edition 1914. A scientific essay for the public and medical profession. First book on Iridology in English in U.S.A.

NILS LILJEQUIST of Stockholm, Sweden. Ministerial Appointee, Anundajo, Sweden. In 1871 published his newly discovered *Quinine and Iodine Change the Color of the Iris. Diagnosis From the Eye — Iridology,* 4th Edition was translated by Dr. J. D. Larson, Iridology Publishing Co., Illinois, Copyright 1916 (English). Liljequist sojourned in United States from October 1, 1914, to February 27, 1915, under sponsorship of Dr. Larson who underwrote travel expense and guaranteed stipulated money for service and instructions.

HENRY LINDLAHR, M.D., was a champion in working with The Healing Crisis. He had a nature cure sanitarium near Chicago, Illinois. His work was based on completely taking care of the whole body. I got my first instruction in *Iridology* from Dr. Lindlahr. He wrote *Irisdiagnosis and Other Diagnostic Methods,* 1st Edition 1919.

DR. BENEDICT LUST of New York and New Jersey. He was a staunch champion of the Water Cure and brought Father Kneipp's water cure method from Europe to the United States. He was a vigorous supporter of Priesnitz and Kuhne, nature cure practitioners, who used water cure in Germany and other parts of Europe.

BERNARR McFADDEN was a great man and respected the muscle structure of the body most. Without exercise and the muscles working properly, he said to me, ''You cannot have good elimination ... nothing in the body will work well without a good muscle structure ... 80 percent of the body depends on the structure of the muscles to carry on the life processes. This includes the bowels and the circulation of blood and lymph in the various parts of the body.'' He was a great walker and made records throughout the country in his walks. He offered many prizes to those who would walk with him.

RICHARD MURRELL McLAIN, D.C., N.D., Los Angeles, California. Born in 1890. Graduated from Los Angeles College of Chiropractic in 1920. Later served as instructor in spinal analysis. Became interested in Iridology in 1926 and taught Iridology from 1929 to 1953 at International School of Professional Arts and Sciences. Also conducted classes in Oregon and has appeared before many Chiropractic and Naturopathic organizations in the United States. Wrote numerous articles on Iridology for publication in professional and laymen's journals. Excellent work done in Iridology research. Dr. McLain was my first teacher and the first man able to demonstrate to me that Iridology was factual and workable.

MARKO J. PETINAK, Ph.D., N.D., D.C., Los Angeles, California. *Eyes in General Diagnosis* published in 1939. 122 pages, 6 x 9''. Iridiology, drug symptoms and signs, visual disorders, pathologies of eyelids, eyeballs and pupil and ophthalmoscopy. Born in what is now Yugoslavia in 1895. Began his Iridology studies as a young man in

VI

Europe and during 1921 and 1922 began preparation of his book *Eyes in General Diagnosis.* Resorted to use of anatomical drawings to illustrate various iris areas related to organs. One of my persoanl teachers. **V.G. ROCINE** was one of the greatest of all teachers that I know. He taught me the biochemical story about the chemicals that are found in our foods and how to make food our medicine and medicine our food. He popularized health cocktails, health salads, health breads and accented inclusion of health ideas in all of our diets and programs. He is the man that developed the 16 chemical types and brought out the Science of Brominosis. He was a Norwegian Homeopath who knew how to get the Homeopathic principles out of food. I have taken many hours in classwork with him.

PETER JOHANNES THIEL of Germany. *Diagnosis of Disease by Observation of the Eye,* 1st Edition in 1905. Translated into English with special notes by Dr. F. W. Collins (1918), Part II of Dr. Collins' book on Iridology 1908-1919.

DR. JOHN H. TILDEN of Denver, Colorado — A great Medical Doctor who emphasized taking care of the ills of mankind by fasting. Trained in medicine but turned to the art of constructive healing by changing people's habits of living. His first step was to eliminate the old through fasting and building a finer functioning body through natural foods and right living methods. He was responsible for many turning to a simple life and a clean way of living. I got my start with fasting with this man.

IGNATZ VON PECZELY of Egervar near Budapest, Hungary. Born January 26, 1826. First and only book published in 1880, *Discovery of Nature and Art of Healing.* His Iris Chart was presented in 1886 by Dr. Zeppritz, Editor of *Homeopathic Monthly Report.* Baginsky placed von Peczely's birth as Monyorokek, Loew, Hungary. Son of the administrator of a Count's estate. About 1857 or 1858 he became interested in Homeopathy. Enrolled in University of Vienna in 1868 where he received his diploma. According to Peczely's grandnephew, Dr. A.S. von Peczely, the birth of Iris Diagnosis is to be placed within the year 1861. Between 1861 and 1880 nothing was heard from von Peczely. In 1873 according to Baginsky, the first edition of von Peczely's book, which founded Iris Diagnosis, was issued. Further manuscripts were not printed and became lost. Von Peczely's work remained unnoticed until 1885 when Zoeppritz procured a treatise on von Peczely's findings.

DR. GEORGE S. WEGER — A Medical Doctor who practiced in Redlands, California. He was one of my teachers and I spent a considerable amount of time with him. He believed in fasting. I saw most unusual cases of chronic diseases successfully handled by his method and I got my fasting knowledge from him while he practiced in Redlands. Published in 1931, *The Genesis and Control of Disease.*

PAUL WERMUTH of Switzerland — A book presenting the history, characteristics and development of Iridology (German), also, *A Glance At Diagnosis From the Eye* (English) based on his own research. (Information received September 1955. Date of publication not given.) Had been using Iridology for the previous 18 years.

DEDICATION

It has been my great pleasure to see this approach of healing unravel in my 50 years of practice. I am very grateful to those patients that have worked with me in this healing method. I want to congratulate those patients who have had the fortitude to carry through all the elimination processes and the healing crisis so that they could have that better health they were seeking ...

Bernard Jensen, D.C., Ph. D.

"Seek not to learn, but to think. Seek not to accept what is told you, but to question..."

"It is a good student who will question what is taught him ... And it is a good professor who, if he is not sure of his ground, will link arms with the student and say, 'Let us go and find out'..."

"Remember that fifteen units of study a semester may eventually lead to a degree, but not necessarily to a real education ... You will find that the mind is not a pail to fill, but a dynamo to start working."

—From a speech by a University President
to a gathering of students.

GET ACQUAINTED WITH THESE TERMS:

Elimination and **Elimination Diets** relate to discharge from the body of indigestible materials and waste products, which is done through five eliminative organs: skin, kidneys, liver, lungs and bowel, and we could add another — the lymphatic system.

Detoxification relates to reduction of toxic materials in the body and making this toxic material easier to be eliminated. So the first part of my health program involves enabling the body to begin rejecting materials collected in the years before from bad diet and poor health habits.

Reversal Process is the retracing of the stages or steps of each disease you have had, reactivating each one and eliminating it. Many people who have suppressed diseases all their lives think an elimination, such as a cold, is a sickness instead of a healing process.

Healing Crisis follows the Reversal Process. It is an effort on all organs to become new and strong again. Though it may feel like a disease crisis, it will not last as long, or develop into another disease. Instead, it will bring about renewed health.

Catarrh, phlegm and **mucus** are a termination process of toxic materials, acid and debris which the body does not want. It can be the end result of the body tissues breaking down and has to find a way out of the body. The accumulation of this material can be eliminated through any orifice, skin or any of the eliminative organs.

CONTENTS

INTRODUCTION

Nature's creative power exceeds man's inclination to destroy.

It should be noted that eighty percent of all diseases in the United States are of a chronic nature. People develop chronic diseases over a period of years, as will be explained later.

I would like to give first a briefing on how my treatments work. To overcome a chronic disease requires right living, good food, and an elimination and detoxification program. In almost all cases I start with detoxification. I like my patients, new and old, to be familiar with elimination diets, detoxification, the reversal process, the healing crisis, and to have a clear understanding of them.

CHAPTER ONE

DEATH BEGINS IN THE COLON

The report *Discussion of Alimentary Toxemia* follows which was given before the Royal Society of Medicine of Great Britain by courtesy of George Lachnicht, Jr., D.C., of Michigan and as covered in the World Iridology Fellowship Journal of December 1974:

"Recently, the subject of alimentary toxemia was discussed in London before the Royal Society of Medicine, by fifty-seven of the leading physicians of Great Britain. Among the speakers were eminent surgeons, physicians and specialists in the various branches of medicine.

"The following is a list of the various poisons of alimentary intestinal toxemia noted by the several speakers: Indol, skatol, phenol, cresol, indican, sulphurretted hydrogen, ammonia, histidine, urrobilin, methylmercaptan, tetramerhy-lendiamin, pentamethy lendiamine, putrescin, cadaverin, neurin, cholin, muscarine, butyric acid, bera-imidazzolethy-lamine, methylgandimine, ptomarropine, botulin, tyramine, agamatine, tryptophane, sepsin, idolethylamine, and sulpher-roglobine. Of these 36 poisons just mentioned, several are highly active, producing most profound effects, and in very small quantities. In cases of alimentary toxemia some one or several of these poisons is constantly bathing the delicate body cells and setting up changes which finally result in a grave disease.

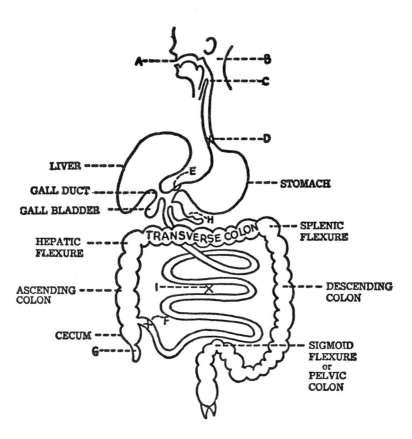

A Mouth Salivary Glands
B Tonsil Cavity
C Esophagus
D Entrance to Stomach
E Duodenum
F Ileo-cecal Valve
G Appendix
H Pancreas
I Approximate Location of
   Umbilicus (Navel)

The alimentary canal, 30 feet in length, consists of the organs of deglutition — the mouth, pharynx, and esophagus; and the organs of digestion — the stomach and the small and large intestines.

"It should be understood that these findings are not mere theories, but are the results of demonstration in actual practice by eminent physicians. Of course, it is not claimed that alimentary toxemia is the only cause of all the symptoms and diseases named; although, of many it may be the sole or principal cause, some of them are due to other causes as well. In the following summary the various symptoms and disorders mentioned in the discussion in London, to which reference has been made above, are grouped and classified."

The Digestive Organs

"Duodenal ulcer causing partial or complete obstruction of the duodenum: pyloric spasm; pyloric obstruction; distension and dilation of the stomach; gastric ulcer; cancer of the stomach; adhesions of the omentum to the stomach and liver; inflammation of the liver; cancer of the liver. The muscular wall of the intestine as well as other muscles atrophies, so that the passage of their contents is hindered. The abdominal viscera lose their normal relationship to the spine and to each other, on account of weakening of the abdominal muscles; these

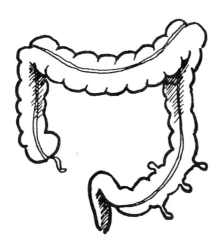

Diverticuli or pockets in the bowel. (From *"Science and Practice of Iridology"* by Dr. Bernard Jensen, D.C.)

displacements are much more marked and serious in women. Other conditions are: catarrh of the intestines; foul gases and foul-smelling stools; colitis; acute enteritis; appendicitis, acute and chronic; adhesions and ''kinks'' of the intestines; visceroptosis; enlargement of the spleen; distended abdomen; tenderness of the abdomen; summer diarrhea in children; inflammation of the pancreas; chronic dragging abdominal pains; gastritis; cancer of the pancreas; inflammatory changes of the gall bladder; cancer of the gall bladder; gallstones; degeneration of the liver; cirrhosis of the liver; infection of the gums, and decay of the teeth; ulcers in the mouth and pharynx.''

Heart and Blood Vessels

''Wasting and weakening of the heart muscles; microbic cyamosis from breaking up of blood cells; fatty degeneration of the heart; endocarditis, myocarditis; subnormal blood pressure; enlargement of the heart; the dilitation of the aorta; high blood pressure; arteriosclerosis; permanent dilation of the arteries. Dr. W. Bezley says: 'There are but a few phases of cardiovascular trouble (disease of heart and blood vessels) with which disorder of some part of the alimentary tract is not causatively associated.'''

The Nervous System

''Headaches of various kinds — frontal, occipital, temporal, dull or intense, hemicranic; headache of a character to lead to a mistaken diagnosis of brain tumor. Dr. Lane tells of a case where a surgeon had proposed an operation for the removal of a tumor from the frontal lobe of the brain; the difficulty was wholly removed by the exclusion of the colon. Acute neuralgia pains in the legs; neuritis; twitching of the eyes and of muscles of the face, arms, legs, etc.; lassitude; irritability; disturbances of the nervous system, varying from simple headaches to absolute collapse; mental and physical depression; insomnia; troubled sleep, unpleasant dreams; unrefreshing sleep, the patient awakening tired; excessive sleepiness, the patient falling asleep in the daytime; shivery sensation across the lower spinal region; burning sensations in the face, hands, etc.; epileptiform tic; typhoid state; paralysis; chronic fatigue; horror of noises; morbid introspection; perverted moral feelings; melancholia, mania, loss of memory; difficulty in mental concentration; imbecility; insanity delirium; coma.''

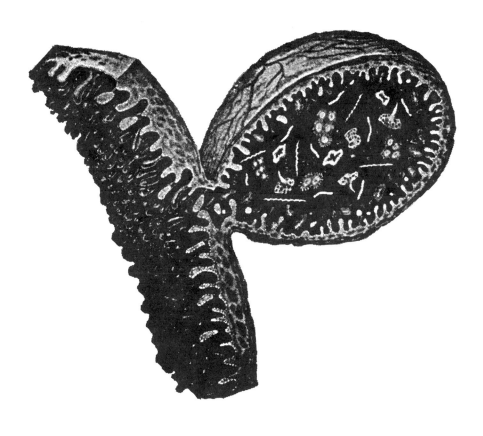

Pocketed conditions in the bowel usually occur as an inherent sickness and it is within these pockets that we have intestinal putrefaction and fermentation developing from this particular part of the colon. Reflex conditions to various organs in the body can develop as the toxious material is picked up from these pockets and carried by the blood to the next weakest organ in the body and usually settles there as a catarrh, phlegm, mucus and to be eliminated by another eliminative organ. (From *"Science and Practice of Iridology"* by Dr. Bernard Jensen, D.C.)

The Eyes

"Degenerative changes in the eye; inflammation of the lens; inflammation of the optic nerve; hardening of the lens; sclerotitis; sclerokeratitis; iritis; iridocyclitis; cataract; recurrent hemmorrhage in the retina; eye dull and heavy."

The Skin

"Formation of wrinkles; thin, inelastic, starchy skin; pigmentations of the skin — yellow, brown, slate-black, blue; muddy complexion; offensive secretion from skin of flexures; thickening of the skin of the back of the skin — sores and boils; pemphigus; pruritus; herpes; eczema; dermatitis; lupus erythemaposus; acne rosacrea; cold, clammy extremeties; dark circles under the eyes; seborrhea; psoriasis; pityriasis; alopecia, lichen; planus; jauncide.

"'An infinitesimal amount of poison may suffice to cause skin eruption.'"

Muscles and Joints

"Degeneration of the muscles: 'Muscles waste and become soft and in advanced cases tear easily.' 'In young life the muscular debility produces the deformities which are called dorsal excurvation, or round shoulders, leteral curvature, flat-foot, and knock-knee.' Weakness of abdominal muscles causes accumulation of feces in the pelvic colon, which renders evacuation of contents more and more difficult. Prominence of bones, rheumatic pains simulating sciatica and lumbago; various muscular pains; muscular rheumatism; arthritis deformities; synavitis; rickets; arthritis, acute and chronic. Tubercle, and rheumatoid arthritis are the direct result of intestinal intoxication. Dr. Lane says: 'I do not believe it is possible for either of these diseases to obtain a foothold except in the presence of stasis.'"

Genito-Urinary and Reproductive Organs

"Various displacements, distortion and disease of the uterus; change in the whole forms contour of woman; fibrosis of breast; wasting of breasts; induration of breasts; sub-acute and chronic mastitis; cancer of breast; merritis and endomestritis; infection of bladder especially in women; frequent urination; albumosuria; acute nephritis; movable kidney; floating kidney. Dr. Lane goes so far as to say: 'Autointoxication plays so large a part in the development of disease of the female genito-urinary apparatus, that they may be regarded by the gynecologist as a product of intestinal stasis.'''

General Disorders and Disturbances of Nutrition

''Degeneration of the organs of elimination, especially the liver, kidneys (Bright's disease) and spleen, pernacious anemia; lowered resistance to infection of all kind; premature senile decay; retardation of growth in children, accompanied by mental irritability and muscular fatigue; adenoids, enlarged tonsils; scurvy; enlarged thyroid (goitre); various tumors and thyroid; Raynaud's disease. In those who apparently suffer no harm from constipation during a long series of years there is perhaps, as suggested by Hertz, a partial immunity established. The writer has long believed that such an immunity is sometimes established in the very obstinate constipation which accompanies absolute fasting, because of the cleansing of the tongue and reappearance of appetite which often occurs at the end of the second or third week of the fast, a phenomenon very like that which appears in typhoid fever and other continued fevers. It must not be supposed, however, that even the establishment of so-called immunity insures the body against all injury. The labor of eliminating an enormous amount of virulent toxins, which falls upon the kidneys, damages the renal tissues and produces premature failure of these essential organs. Any process which develops toxins within the body is a menace to the life of the tissues and should be suppressed as far as possible, and as quickly as possible.

''The fact that symptoms of poisoning resulting from constipation do not appear at once is no evidence that injury is not done. Dr. William Hunter in the course of the London discussion remarked that the fact that chronic constipation 'might exist in certain individuals as an almost permanent condition without apparently causing ill health is due solely to the power and protective action of the liver. It is not any evidence of the comparative harmlessness of constipation per se, but only an evidence that some individuals possess the cecum and the colon of an ox, with the liver of a pig, capable of doing any amount of distoxication.' In the face of such an array of evidence backed up by authority of nearly 60 eminent English physicians — and many hundreds of other English, U.S., German and French physicians whose names might be added — it is no longer possible to ignore the importance of alimentary toxemia or autointoxication as a fact in the production of disease. To no other single cause is it possible to attribute one-tenth as many various and widely diverse disorders. It may be said that almost every chronic disease known is directly or indirectly due to the influence of bacterial poisons absorbed from the intestine. The colon may be justly looked upon as a veritable Pandora's box, out of which come more human misery and suffering, mental and moral, as well as physical than from any other known source.

''The colon is a sewage system, but by neglect and abuse it becomes a cesspool. When it is clean and normal we are well and happy; let it stagnate, and it will distill the poisons of decay, fermentation and putrefaction into the blood, poisoning the brain and nervous system so that we become mentally depressed and irritable; it will poison the heart so that we are weak and listless; poisons the lungs so that the breath is foul; poisons the digestive organs so that we are distressed and bloated; and poisons the blood so that the skin is sallow and unhealthy. In short, every organ of the body is poisoned, and we age prematurely, look and feel old, the joints are stiff and painful, neuritis, dull eyes and a sluggish brain overtake us; the pleasure of living is gone.

''The preceding information should impress you with the vital importance of bowel regularity to you and every member of your family.''

CHAPTER TWO

AUTOINTOXICATION

Autointoxication is defined as: ''The poisoning of the body, or some part of the body, by toxic matter generated therein.''

The following appeared in the *World Iridology Fellowship Journal* of December 1974, on the subject of autointoxication resulting from intestinal putrefaction and the finding of INDICAN — a byproduct of putrefaction — in urine:

''Stedman's Medical Dictionary: Indican — the mother substance of indigo-blue, a yellowish or colorless syrupy glucoside; or indoxyl sulphate, a substance found in the sweat and in variable amount in urine.

''Indicanuria: The presence in excess in the urine of indican, derived from indole produced in protein putrefaction in the intestine and in putrefactive changes elsewhere. (Indican = Indoxyl potassium sulphate). In gallstone attacks, in hyperchlorhydris, in recurring appendicitis, in wasting diseases, in peritonitis, and in empyemia, it is usually present, in a few cases it is constant.

''The enzymes in and produced by micro-organisms in the intestine, break down some of the undigested polysaccharides, proteins and other complex compounds. Comment has been made that the end products from carbohydrate breakdown are usually innocuous, whereas many of the compounds resulting from the decomposition of protein are toxic.

The latter fact has given rise to the assumption that when the rate of production and absorption of these products is increased above normal as in constipation, a condition of autointoxication is produced, which is characterized by malaise, headache, irritability and other symptoms.

"It should be borne in mind that no trace of indican may, or may not, be indicative of the absence of putrefaction. In the absence of putrefaction a negative reading would be expected, but a single test cannot be relied upon. Experience has shown that a **restored** efficiency of the manifold eliminative processes may **increase** excretion of indican and this would be indicative of **retention** of the products of putrefaction previously.''

Consider the average person walking down the street ... chances are he or she is at least half sick. We think of the man who fell out of a 20-story window. As he passed the second story window, he remarked, "Well, I'm all right so far!" So it is with people living dangerously, partaking of poisoning foods. They may be "all right so far," but how long will it last?

Unfortunately, many people living dangerously do not realize what they are doing. They continue to drink alcoholic beverages or beverages loaded with other toxic poisons, smoke tobacco, overeat and partake of foods difficult to digest such as white bread or foods containing white sugar. They just do not understand the effects of bad food, smoking and drinking habits. They do not know, for instance, that a shortage of natural fresh foods in the diet will create a shortage of enzymes and a corresponding increase in the work of the enzyme-producing glands. For example, a food such as papaya has a considerable quantity of enzymes. By eating this food and other foods containing enzymes, they can avoid over-working the pancreas. The pancreas produces juices needed in digestion. It also produces insulin, needed to control carbohydrates. Insufficient ingestion of natural foods, combined with excessive use of foods requiring large amounts of pancreatic juices such as white bread and sugar, causes the pancreas to work overtime and to become disabled and under-produce the necessary juices. Insufficient enzymes are said to cause degenerative disease. Why take a chance?

People do not know the effects of tobacco on the system. They have never seen, as this writer has seen, smoke blown into a bottle and the smoke then adhere to the sides of the bottle. As Dr. Melchior T. Dikkers, has pointed out in his book "Unintentional Suicide," smoking causes the mucous membranes to become chronically inflammed and consequently more easily penetrated by exhaust gases in the air and this is a direct causative factor in the production of cancer.

People also do not know that alcohol destroys important nutrients and this causes vitamin deficiencies and mineral imbalances. There is particularly a shortage created in Vitamin B1 (thiamine) and nicotinic acid (niacin). In addition, autopsies reveal that the brain of the alcoholic shrinks and brain power is reduced. Alcohol slows down reflex actions, perception, judgment and speech. Eyesight suffers and muscular coordination is greatly reduced. Why should one poison oneself with alcohol?

Autointoxication is self-poisoning ... which is slow suicide. When done through ignorance, it is unintentional suicide. When done because of stubborness, it is intentional suicide. Life can and should be sweet and wonderful. Why shorten it by suicide?

Laxatives

As a rule, I do not believe in laxatives. Laxatives are usually of an irritable nature and the body wants to get rid of this irritation and produces an increased peristaltic action to get rid of the impacted material. There are times when a laxative can be used to a good advantage but it should be of a temporary nature.

The greatest thing that I have found to help the bowel and to help along the inactivity of inherent weaknesses within the bowel itself where there is poor tone, where there is a stagnant condition in any part of the bowel, where the muscle structure has lost its tone many times caused from sedentary occupations and can be even an inherent weakness, is ... Alfalfa Tablets. Alfalfa is the greatest thing I have found for the care of the bowel. This is made up of the fiber or the bulk of the leaf of the alfalfa. This gives the weakened bowel tissue something to exercise on and it gradually becomes stronger. It is a food and it has nourishing qualities so the compensation that you get from it is a building one. The chlorophyll found in Alfalfa Tablets helps to develop the friendly bacteria, getting rid of odorous gases and is a good food for the intestinal flora or the friendly acidopholus bacteria. We give four on an average to each person for each meal. Crack them once before swallowing them. Take them right along with the meal and in between bites of food as you desire. The chlorophyll also helps to sustain the bowel.

CHAPTER THREE

ELIMINATION DIETS

There are many things to be used in detoxifying the bowel. The best thing to do is to go on an eleven day elimination diet as shown below. That means starting with a fast for a day or two, drinking a half glass of water every hour and a half or so. Then drink juices for two or three days, fruits and vegetables for a few days, and then fruits and vegetables along with cooked foods. At the end of eleven days, you are ready to go to the regular diet again. This is a good program to start with:

Eleven Day Elimination Regime

There are many eliminative regimes and they all accomplish about the same results through the fact that the body is given less food, simpler foods and simpler combinations, more watery food ... a greater transition can take place in the cells of the body.

This Eleven Day Elimination Regime can be used by most persons in health and for those who want to overcome the average physical disorder. Those who are weak or feeble, however, should not follow the plan the full eleven days without supervision. Those with tuberculosis should have both supervision and assistance.

Variation as to the length of time and the manner in which the foods are to be taken may be adjusted to suit the history and activities of the patient. Examples: fruits, vegetables and broths can be taken for one or, one day of just fruit, or, one, two or three days of vegetables only.

Vegetables taken in the form of broths, gently steamed vegetables and salads are a safer routine for the average beginner than citrus fruits.

A hot bath should be taken every night during this diet regime. Enemas may be used the first four or five days, then discontinued for natural movements. Nothing but water and fruit juices, preferably grapefruit, should be taken into the body for the first three days. Drink one glass of juice every four hours of the day. The next two days fruit only — such as grapes, melons, tomatoes, pears, peaches, plums, or dried fruit such as prunes, figs, peaches, soaked overnight, and baked apple.

In the six following days breakfast should consist of citrus fruits. Between breakfast and lunch any other kind of fruit. For a lunch have a salad of three to six vegetables and two cups of vital broth. When hungry between meals, fruit or fruit juices may be taken. Dinner should consist of two or three steamed vegetables and two cups of vital broth. Fruit juices can be taken before retiring if wanted.

Rigid adherence to the diet is an absolute necessity for anyone attempting to regain good health. Eat plenty but not to satisfy.

Vital Broth Recipe:

½ C. carrot tops
2 C. potato peeling (½ inch thick)
2 C. beet tops
2 C. celery tops
3 C. celery stalk
2 qts. distilled water
½ tsp. Savita or Vegex
Add a carrot and onion to flavor if desired (grate or chop)

Ingredients should be finely chopped. Bring to a boil slowly, simmer approximately 20 minutes. Use only the broth after straining.

When finished with the above regime return to Dr. Jensen's Daily **Food Regime.**

The above elimination regime should be followed whenever a person changes from the old ways of living and begins to live right. As a rule it is wise to follow the elimination regime in any and all of the following cases: As a General Cleanser two or three times a year; at a time of crisis; when reduction of weight is desired; when hips get too large; when joints get stiff; when the skin breaks out; when constipation is present.

Remember that vegetables can also be detoxifying. The greatest vegetables for use in bowel problems are summer squash, zucchini and yellow crooked neck squash . . . they are the best for the bowel. In parts of Europe banana squash is used, baked, and makes a wonderful, soothing food for the bowel. All fruits and vegetables that are yellow are laxative. So take care of the bowel first with green and yellow foods.

The Grape Diet presented in a following page is a detoxifying diet. The Eleven Day Elimination Diet and the Grape Diet can be used beautifully and still allow you to work, exercise and take hikes and walks. They enable you to keep going, so you can keep up with other people. You may be on it while working, however, it is best to rest as much as possible.

Fasting

Fasting is the quickest way of bringing about elimination in the body and the fastest way of getting toxic materials out of the body. This is done through complete rest . . . physical, psychological and psychic.

As we let the body rest, it develops tone and vitality, more than is possible by any other procedure. I believe rest is a cure because it gives us the vitality we need to throw off toxic material and to eliminate the debris that has been accumulated over a period of years. We can literally withdraw toxic accumulations through a fast. We find that there are many ways to fast. I think the better way is to take a half glass of water every hour and a half throughout the day. If it is a hot day you may need water and it is all right since you perspire more. Be sure not to take big gulps of water at one time. The water should be cool and not ice cold.

Take daily enemas the first few days, then reduce this to every other day or every third or fourth day, depending upon the length of time you fast. While you are fasting you should rest as much as possible. If you hike or walk, do it on level ground. Do nothing to the point of tiring.

This is important in fasting.

Breaking A Fast:

In breaking a fast, the best way to do this is to go remember that if you go five, six or seven days on water, then go one or two days on juices, either vegetable or fruit. Take one 8 ounce glass every three hours. You have eliminated the enemas one or two days beforehand and you are starting in to work for good bowel movements now.

After the two days of juices, start the first thing in the morning on the third day with sliced or peeled oranges. The bulk of an orange is probably one of the finest things for the bowel. If you do not want to use oranges, you can use a finely shredded carrot that has been steamed or wilted for one minute or a minute and a half to just wilt it. This acts to help clean out the toxic materials. You can do this for breakfast and lunch. Then for the evening meal you can start out with a small salad. Have a glass of juice at 10:00 A.M. and again at 3:00 P.M.

The next day you can have fresh fruit for breakfast along with juice. Have juice at 10:00 A.M. For lunch you can have a small salad and juice. Have another glass of juice at 3:00 P.M.

At the evening meal you can have a salad, one cooked vegetable and juice.

The next day you can have the same as the day before, except that you could have an extra vegetable at noon and again at night if desired. You could probably also have an egg, or a tablespoon of nut butter, for the morning meal.

The next day, you will start on Dr. Jensen's Regular Diet, except for no starches.

The day following, you can have both starches and proteins in your diet.

****

If you go on a 14 day Water Fast, it is well that you consider going three days on juices before starting in on foods again. Hoever, it is not necessary. You can almost do the same as when breaking the 7 day Water Fast, but if you go to 21 days, you must be sure to stay at least the three days on juices before eating food.

If you are taking enemas through these days, make sure you stop all enemas three or four days before you start eating solid foods. Start working for natural bowel movements again.

And remember ... no supplements on the fasting program.

One Day A Week Fast

On a one day a week fast regime you can be on a juice diet or a fruit on the one day ... and rest. Many people like to go on a fast one day a week. This is perfectly all right if you will rest that day ... but you MUST rest! You cannot expect to get the good yielded by a rest without food by using all of your energy and leaving yourself depleted by working on a day that you do not eat.

Bulks

There are many diets that can include bulk. There are many bulks in the market, for example, Metamucil, Sonne #7 and Sonne #9, Deturge, Serutan. All of these can be purchased in health food stores. Follow directions. You may find that to begin with you will have to use laxative foods to move the bulk along. Or it may be desirable to take faxseed tea enemas, as mentioned in a following page.

Sonne #7 is Bentonite, a clay, and Sonne #9 is a bulk. When used with the eleven day elimination diet, it makes for the best elimination diet I know.

We must watch for impactions in the bowel and sometimes bulk furthers these impactions. A lazy bowel many times does not move bulk along very well. It may need massage and enema to help remove it.

There are many different kinds of diets and it might be well to realize that just taking a fruit breakfast every day will help you to reduce and to detoxify the body.

Our *Healthy Way To Live* diet is half eliminating and detoxifying and half building.

Extra juices in the diet will also help to eliminate. This can be done at 10:00 in the morning and/or at 3:00 in the afternoon.

Get OFF Of That Diet ... It is very important to realize that what we are giving you are diets that can eliminate, can reduce, can get rid of toxic material but they are still diets. And there are so many people that are on a diet all the time and eliminating all the time. They never have any food building materials going into the body nor are they following a balanced way of eating. This is why we have included our healthy way of living. You must get OFF of diets and back to a healthy way of living. That is not only in foods but in exercise and so forth.

It is well to consult the patient's handbook *Creating A Magic Kitchen*. It was developed to help the patient set up the proper kitchen and the correct way of living to get the most out of the pantry and the kitchen that should be serving us good health.

Working to produce a crisis in the body is very important. However, you don't have to do it immediately. When a person comes under our care, we work for this as soon as possible ... we work according to the patient's activities, job, and consciousness. You can come to a crisis by following a healthy way to live, and especially so, if you have been living on coffee and donuts, pickles and ice cream. Our healthy way of living is a great step up from that type of living. When you give up junk foods and come into this way of life, your body automatically molds into what you eat and how you live. So a crisis will develop of its own accord. The reversal process has already started the moment that you add the herb teas and more of the fruits and vegetables to your diet.

The Master Chlorophyll Elimination Diet

This is a diet of just plain water, preferable using distilled water, and using one teaspoon of a liquid chlorophyll to one glass of water every three hours. You can also use vegetable juice, but this is a diet where we are adding iron, gathering all the oxygen we can while we are breathing, and burning up the toxic waste by using the iron as found in liquid chlorophyll. Liquid chlorophyll is usually made as an extract from alfalfa leaves, which is one of the highest things we have in potassium iron, which will attract the oxygen to the body. Doing this for three or four days is a wonderful pre-elimination diet to fasting or to any other type of dieting. I consider this to be the master-cleansing diet for all catarrhal conditions. In the presence of greens, we find that catarrh is eliminated best from the body.

****

There are a couple of **Reducing Diets** that we would like to include here. One is for the vegetarian and one for the meat-eater. I will say that those who go on the meat reducing diet will find that it will take off weight best of all. We have used both diets for some years and find that they really do take the weight off.

We usually go one week on the reducing diet, one week on the regular diet, one week on the reducing diet, and one week on the regular diet. We alternate for a period of two months. This way we can see that we lose on the reducing diet and probably hold our weight on the regular diet.

There is an extreme elimination diet placed at the bottom of the meat diet if you would like to lose in a hurry and would like to get off more weight as you go along.

REDUCING DIET

Follow this diet for _____ weeks. Then, return to Dr. Jensen's Regular Diet for _____ weeks. (Back to the Reducing Diet for _____ weeks).

□□□□□□□□

The meats used may be lamb, fish, lean beef, turkey, chicken. We never have fats or pork. Bake, broil or roast fish and meat. The fish should be a white fish (one that has fins and scales).

Always use tomato (sliced, ripe) (canned in emergency) or grapefruit when you eat meat or fish.

If you do not use meat, then use the other proteins: eggs, cottage cheese, gelatin mold, skim milk, soy milk, soy tofu, lo-fat yogurt.

All vegetables should be from the 5% Carbohydrate List outlined below.

Drink in-between meals, **only**. This should be one hour before, or two hours after meals. Use KB-11 or Cleaver tea (2 cups daily).

5% CARBOHYDRATE VEGETABLES

Artichokes	Chicory	Mustard Greens	String Beans
Asparagus	Cucumber	Okra	Swiss Chard
Beet Greens	Dandelion	Radishes	Tomatoes
Broccoli	Eggplant	Rhubarb	Turnip Tops
Brussel Sprouts	Endive	Sauerkraut (not canned)	Vegetable Marrow
Cabbage	Escarole	Sea Kale	Watercress
Cauliflower	Leeks	Sorrel	
Celery	Lettuce	Sprouts (alfalfa, mung, etc.)	
Chard	Mushroom	Spinach	

REGULAR REDUCING DIET

Suggested Eating Plan for a week:

BREAKFAST: Fresh Fruit (1) and 1 or 2 Eggs or Cottage Cheese.
LUNCH: Brown Rice and 1 Vegetable and Salad.
DINNER: Meat or Fish with tomato or grapefruit, and 1 Vegetable (if desired).

OTHER MEAL SUGGESTIONS
FOR REGULAR REDUCING DIET

1. Skim Milk, 1 tablespoon of Sesame Seed Meal, ⅓ Avocado and 1 Fruit. Liquefy.
2. Skim Milk, watercress or romaine lettuce (liquefy) and Salad with Fish and Tomato.
3. Skim Milk, watercress or romaine lettuce (liquefy) and Salad with Fish and Tomato.
4. Fruit and Cheese
5. Apples and Cottage Cheese.
    You may use Rice Cakes or Rye Crisp once in awhile.

STRICT REDUCING DIET

Only use this Menu:

BREAKFAST: Fresh Fruit (1) and 1 or 2 Eggs.
LUNCH: Vegetable and Salad.
DINNER: Meat or Fish with tomato or grapefruit.

VEGETARIAN REDUCING DIET

Follow this diet for _____ weeks. Then, return to Dr. Jensen's Regular Diet
for _____ weeks. Back to Reducing Diet for _____ weeks.

□□□□□□□□

VEGETARIAN REGULAR REDUCING DIET

Suggested Eating Plan for a Week:

BREAKFAST: Fresh Fruit (1) and 1 or 2 Eggs or Cottage Cheese
LUNCH: Brown Rice and Vegetable (1) and Salad.
DINNER: Protein (see list) with tomato or grapefruit, and Vegetable (1), if desired.

———————

Other Meal Suggestions:

1. Soy Milk or Skim Milk, 1 tablespoon of Sesame Seed Meal, ⅓ Avocado and 1 fruit. Liquefy.
2. Fruit and Cheese.
3. Apple and Lo-Fat Yogurt.
4. Skim Milk, watercress or romaine lettuce (liquefy); Salad with Fish and Tomato (or, use 4-6 watercress tablets per meal).
   You may use Rice Cakes or Rye Crisp once in awhile.

———————

VEGETARIAN STRICT REDUCING DIET

BREAKFAST: Fresh Fruit (1) and 1 or 2 Eggs.
LUNCH: Vegetable Salad.
DINNER: Protein with Tomato or Grapefruit.

———————

BOTH VEGETARIAN DIETS:
  Drink in-between meals **only**. This should be at least one hour before or two hours after meals. Use KB 11 or Cleaver Tea (2 cups daily).

BOTH VEGETARIAN DIETS:
  Use tomato (sliced, ripe) (or canned in emergency) or grapefruit with proteins at Dinner.

PROTEINS: Fish, Eggs, Cottage Cheese, Gelatin Mold, Soy Tofu, Lo-Fat Yogurt. (Fish used should be one that had fins and scales.)

———————

BOTH VEGETARIAN DIETS: All vegetables should be from the **5% Carbohydrate List** outlined on previous page.

WARNING

In my opinion it is very difficult to retrace and do a good job in tubercular cases. There has been a breakdown in the calcium control and calcium metabolism and while these cases have gone usually through a suppression, I think it is well not to awaken it again and bring it to the elimination stage. However, a person can go on to fairly good health by living a sensible life by keeping away from the extremes as we take many people through in the elimination diets. Also, diabetes and hypoglycemia must be watched very closely and should be under supervision.

The Carrot Juice Diet

Again let me tell you that carrot juice only, taking it constantly, is a diet. The time comes when you must get off of it because it will not sustain life forever. It is not a perfect food. It is not well balanced and hasn't got all the minerals, vitamins, oils, fats and proteins necessary for building a completely new body. Tissue that needs protein will not get enough of it from the carrots.

Following the carrot juice diet, you can have a gallon to a gallon and a half a day, if you would like, and have a glass of juice regularly every hour or hour and a half during the day.

Sometimes using the enemas that were given beforehand can be used here also.

Some people can go onto the carrot juice diet for a period of a week, some can go two weeks, some a month without any trouble. But we find that it is best to go under these diets, again, with the care of a doctor or your physician.

Carrot Juice

Mary C. Hoegler of Salt Lake City claimed she cured herself of a malignancy and used carrot juice to do this. Mrs. Ferrara out in Monrovia claimed she cured herself with carrot juice. Johanna Bryant said that grapes cured her malignancy.

I don't think it's any particular juice that will cure anything ... but I believe the rest you give your body allows it the opportunity to reverse the disease and recover your health. It's the rest from food and the simple diet that does the trick. The lack of too many food mixtures and less demand made on our digestive and eliminative system helps us to overcome disease.

The carrot juice diet involves taking one glass of carrot juice every three hours or more if you like. You can do this for ten days, twenty days, or even longer. I had one man on carrot juice for a full year. That is a long time! This particular man lived in Monrovia and had an extreme condition of the bowel but through the carrot juice diet he got rid of it.

Dr. Kirshner, who wrote the book on juice therapy, came here to talk over this man's case because he found out how I had kept him on juices for so long a time. The man passed off mucus and catarrh continually from that bowel. It was almost unbelievable what was eliminated ... being even black at times. This was simply accumulated toxic material that was necessary for him to get rid of.

Grapes

Four pounds of grapes a day is a good amount for a grape diet and you should average a pound or so every three hours. These grapes should be the grapes that have seeds since these are the most vital of all grapes. Man has gone to using hybrid foods too much. Those foods that were brought to us in the beginning are the foods that have lots of seeds. They are the vital foods. So, I believe the grapes that have seeds are the best. The Concord, Fresno Beauty, Red grapes and Muscat, all are good grapes to use. I don't say that you have to use the seeds. You can chew them fine if you like. A good thing to help eliminate catarrh is found in cream of tartar which surround the seeds. So make sure you get all the material off the seeds when you are eating them. When chewing grape skins, you'll find that they are very bitter but that bitterness is high in potassium. Potassium is a great cleanser in the body. Gayelord Hauser made his name with potassium broth. It is a great cleanser and detoxifier in the body.

Especially in the beginning of the grape diet, I think you should use enemas. Toxic materials accumulate and it is well that we keep things moving along. You can go on grapes five to ten days without any supervision, but if you stay on them longer, it is well to have someone around that has been used to giving the grape diet. That person should be able to take care of you with any reaction you might have that may be strange to you ... many times these reactions are nothing more than a healing crisis or an elimination process.

Watermelon Flush

There are times during the watermelon season that we can use watermelon as a good elimination diet. Going on watermelon for three, four or five days is a wonderful kidney eliminant, a diuretic. We find that it helps to take out a lot of the debris in the colon and the extra water picks up toxic materials and carries them off.

Potato Peeling Broth

Potato peeling broth is a high potassium broth and is one of the best broths I know for taking care of extreme acids in the body, and especially, rheumatic and arthritic acids. Taking two cups a day for one month, or even two months, in between meals, is tolerated by the average person along with their regular diet. We find that this helps to neutralize acids that have been accumulated over long periods of time. It helps to get rid of the toxic wastes that have settled into various parts of the body and to neutralize the acids that attack the joints. We find that it is a wonderful aid in getting rid of rheumatic pains in the body. This broth can be used right along with a good, healthy way of living.

My Crisis Broth

I find the thing really to do in the time of a crisis is to lean toward the vegetable kingdom. The body is going through an extreme elimination process and sometimes taking too much of the fruit juices forces this elimination more than I think is necessary. I put most of my people on Potato Peeling Broth who go through the healing crisis from one to three days. We lose potassium salts in our body through the elimination process. We replace this with this potassium Potato Peeling Broth.

Herb Teas

Any of the herb teas are helpful. Think of their value and try to relate them to the particular problem you have.

For instance . . . for weak kidneys, there is no reason why you should not use Shave Grass tea, Parsley tea, or kidney and bladder teas available from the health food stores.

A good eliminating tea for kidney structure is made from Juniper berries . . . mash them, pour a cup of hot water on them and let stand until the boiling water is just slightly warm and drink the excellent tea. You may add a little honey if you wish. Using this three times in 24 hours makes this a wonderful kidney detoxifier. You can also cook some fresh asparagus in water and take a half teacup of the water three times a day.

Peppermint tea is good for stomach trouble as well as Camomile tea.

If you have lung catarrh, Comfrey tea and Fenugreek tea may be used two or three times daily.

Flaxseed tea for eliminating toxic materials in the bowel is one of the great elimination and healing factors for the bowel. It is found useful for inflammation or irritations of the bowel, as well as for stomach ulcers.

Steep one teaspoon of flaxseed in a cup of hot water and let stand until it becomes somewhat "mucilaginous". In some cases it is desirable to drink the liquid and discard the seed.

It is of good use in enemas. Some people find that taking plain water enemas is irritating to the bowel but by using a combination of one pint of flaxseed tea and one teaspoon of liquid chlorophyll, they are able to get good results without disturbance or pain. This can be used daily if indicated.

There are other detoxifying diets which can be used. One for instance is cleansing the gallbladder with beet juice or beet juice plus a little olive oil if you wish. There are many detoxifying ideas in the herb category and you should use the many herbs that can be used for your particular condition.

Remember too . . . that we want to get to the place where we use everything possible to build up tissues so they will eliminate toxic substances.

When we mention that it is not well to be on an alkalinizing diet continually and that we may produce an over-alkalinization through these diets, we recognize that this can be an abnormal condition in the body. Proteins and starches added to the diet keeps us from becoming over-alkalinized. The urine is supposed to be acid. If it has become alkaline, it is a sign many times that we are living on too many fruits and vegetbles. While Dr. Jarvis used a tablespoon of apple cider vinegar in a glass of water to bring the urine back to normal, we believe the greatest correction comes when we change our diet habits.

Kneipp Leg Baths

Go outside where you can stand on grass or sand. Take water hose, without spray attachment, and starting from the toes go up the right leg to the groin, then around to back of right leg and down right leg to the heel. Repeat on left leg from toes to groin, around to back of thigh and down left leg to heel. Do each leg only one time up and down and do only one time each day. Do not dry with towel. Walk on sand or grass until legs and feet are dry or approximately ten minutes. Drying with towel would lose the beneficial effect.

You can make a sanitarium out of your home. Your circulation methods are enhanced by using the Kneipp Leg Baths, the Grass Walk,

Sand Walk and walking in the hills to quicken your breath. This enables you to have a quicker elimination of toxic materials demonstrated by bad breath, the body odors through perspiration. We find there is a constant exchange of old tissues for the new. Sleeping at night with a good ventilation in your room is necessary. Above all ... talk about some of the more positive things in life and don't sit at the table talking about your problems and troubles ... especially if they are financial! Never talk about your financial problems while you are eating. Of course, if somebody leaves you a million dollars, then you can talk about it!

Educational programs should be instituted and we should get into bee culture, fish culture and flower culture. Get out in the garden, grow flowers and develop a sense of meaning in your mind. Walk through a flower garden before you go to work in the morning. Don't look at anyone in the morning before you look at flowers! Then you'll never have anything but good to say to whomever you meet. Yes, we have to learn how to unfold our innate good ... how to unfold our soul qualities that are also good for our bodies.

The human body is a servant to the mind ... and ... to the spirit. If you want a good body, you should develop the desire for one.

You have the ideal now, so start pinning up in your mind an idea of the picture of good health you want. Then start singing for it ... whistling for it and living for it.

As soon as you start the detoxification process and begin putting your mind in good order, you will realize that you are on your way to building a strong body. I know it's hard to live the perfect life. But you'll find that as you take on the more Godly ways and the nature cure course, this can outmatch any problem you may have. Remember ... that every problem is always Divinely outmatched!

EXERCISES

We do everything possible to improve elimination, for example, exercise develops tone in tissues and strong tissues eliminate better. So one thing helps the other.

Playful recreation is good and when I speak of this I mean water exercises, baseball, handball, hiking and basketball, to name just a few. They detoxify the body. This induces sweating and promotes circulation of blood and lymph through the tissues and quickens the elimination of toxic waste and rebuilding of cell structure. There are bed exercises that you may have to get acquainted with if you cannot get out and run, jump or jog. There are exercises which can be used under all conditions . . . in open air, in water and even bed exercises such as isometrics. You have to be almost completely ossified not to exercise.

Muscular exercise such as tension and relaxation, and pushing and pulling neck exercises are most important in detoxifying. This form of exercise helps the lymph glands around the neck. Don't forget the midsection exercises for the bowels.

There are liver exercises such as twisting, bending down and turning the body from side to side. There are slanting board exercises. Bring the legs up to the chest, squeezing the abdominal muscles. Try doing the bicycle upside down in bed or on the slanting board. Detoxification also takes place in sunshine. You could have a helio gym, so to speak, where you can do exercises in the nude if possible.

Jumping and rope skipping are wonderful in helping to detoxify the body. You should also investigate the EZE Jogger. This is a great instrument to use if you can't run, jump or walk much.

Rowing in a boat is wonderful for the lung structure and the chest. Bicycling is wonderful for the legs. Consider horseback exercises. They help the stomach, bowel, liver and the circulation. And, of course, consider the social side of your nature.

We are constantly developing a sanitarium. around us by going through this detoxifying program. Sleep is necessary for good detoxification. Try getting to bed early a few nights. I've seen people with swollen ankles that wouldn't respond much to many of the treatments but having them go to bed early and lie prone has helped greatly.

The Value of Exercises in the Reversal Process

It is necessary to have good blood for the repair and rebuilding of good tissue but this tissue must also have tone. I believe that food alone is not the cure in all that we need in the Reversal Process. I advise different exercises especially for the bowel and the abdominal organs to build up the tone that they may function better. A tired, flabby bowel cannot eliminate well, therefore, build up the tone through corrective exercises. The exercises that are best for the abdominal tract are:

Chest Leg Pull Up Exercise which is sitting on the edge of the chair with your shoulders almost touching the back of the chair and the heels almost touching the floor while your hands grasp the side of the chair. Lift the knees to the chest, straighten out the legs but do not touch the floor, bring the legs back and forth for two or three times and up to 10 to 15 times, as you are capable.

The Alley Cat Exercise is another exercise. While standing, lift one leg bending the knee and bringing it in front of the other leg up to the abdomen. Do this with the other leg and do this exercise 10 to 15 times.

The Rubber Ball Exercise is a wonderful exercise while lying in bed using a ball like a tennis ball or handball and rubbing it around the abdomen 25 times beginning on the right side and going completely around in a circle over the abdomen.

Slanting Board Exercises will help all pocketed lazy bowels. It's a great help in prolapsus, colon stasis, gases and regenerating the vital Nerve Center of the brain. I do not believe in using the Slanting Board when there is high blood pressure, (over 185 Systolic), heart disease, internal bleeding, hemorrhages or wherever exercises of any kind are contra-indicated for any abdominal problem.

When there is a lack of tone in the muscles we can expect prolapsus of the abdominal organs. The heart, lacking tone, cannot circulate blood properly throughout the body. Likewise, arteries and veins can not contract to help the blood against gravity into the brain tissues.

There are some people who apparently have tried everything to get well, who still find all organs working under par. Many people do not realize that all the quickening force for every organ of the body comes from the brain. People whose occupations require them to sit or stand continually are unable to get the blood into the brain tissues because the tired organs cannot force the blood uphill. If we deny the brain tissues good blood in the proper amount, in time, every organ in our body will suffer.

The heart gets its start from the brain and continues its everlasting pumping because of it. No organ can do without the brain. I attribute the success of my healing work to the very fact that I definitely recognize that the brain must be fed properly. Slanting board exercises are absolutely necessary to regaining perfect health.

The reports are phenomenal as to what can be done in cases of prolapsus and lack of tone in the abdominal walls. A Mr. C.M. Pierce, who became interested in this form of exercise, has done wonders in rejuvenating his body. We quote from Health News of September 26th, 1941: "One night three years ago I saw Dr. Jensen demonstrate the slanting board and instantly saw how to make my system much easier, and on the way home I told my neighbor, 'I am going to make a board like that.'" Since then he has made many, selling them throughout the country. In fact, Mr. Pierce, who was born October 11, 1866 is still active in his business.

There are many cases where the board is contra-indicated. It is best in most cases to get professional advice, for some people have had unhappy experiences due to the very fact they started too strenuous a program to begin with. If you haven't done much exercising of the abdominal muscles, it is well to take these exercises slowly and gradually increase them as you get stronger.

Do not use the board in cases of high blood pressure, hemorrhages, some tubercular conditions, cancer in the pelvic cavity, appendicitis, ulcers of the stomach or intestines, pregnancy, unless under the care of a physician.

The slanting board exercises are practically the same as any other lying-down exercises. The most important exercise is to hold on to the sides of the board bringing the knees up to the chest. This forces all the abdominal organs up toward the shoulders. While in this position, twist the head from side to side and in all directions, thus utilizing the extra force to circulate blood to congested areas of the head, especially bringing the stomach and abdominal organs up toward the chest while holding the breath.

Slanting board exercises are especially good in cases of imflammations and congestions above shoulders, such as sinus trouble, bad eyes, falling hair, head eczema, ear conditions and similar troubles. Slanting board exercise is needed and has helped more than any other treatment in cases of heart trouble, fatigue, dizziness, poor memory and paralysis. The average person should maintain the foot end of the board at chair height for all exercises, but if dizzy at first, the foot end of the board should not be raised quite so high to begin with. Exercise only five minutes a day if more . . . it is too much. Gradually increase time spent on board. The average patient should lie on the board ten minutes at three o'clock in the afternoon and again just before going to bed. After retiring lift the buttocks up to allow the organs to return to a normal position.

Use Ankle Straps While Doing the Following Exercises

1. Lie full length allowing gravity to help the abdominal organs into their proper position. For results lie on board at least ten minutes.
2. While lying flat on back, stretch the abdomen by putting arms above head. Bring arms above head 10 to 15 times; this stretches the abdominal muscles and pulls the abdomen down toward the shoulders.
3. Bring abdominal organs toward shoulders while holding breath. Move the organs back and forth by drawing them upward, then allowing them to go back to a relaxed position. Do 10 to 15 times.
4. Pat abdomen vigorously with open hands. Lean to one side then to the other, patting the stretched side. Pat 10 to 15 times.
5. Bring the body to sitting, using the abdominal muscles. Return to lying position. Do 3 or 4 times if possible. Do only if Doctor orders.

Hold on the Handles, Feet out of Straps, While Doing These

6. Bend knees and legs at hips. While in this position; (a) turn head from side to side five or six times; (b) lift the head slightly and rotate in circles three or four times.
7. Lift legs to vertical position, rotate outward in circles eight or ten times. Increase to 25 times after a week or two of exercising.
8. Bring legs straight up to a vertical position and lower them to board slowly. Repeat three or four times. Bicycle legs in air 15 to 25 times.
9. Relax and rest, letting the blood circulate in the head for 10 minutes.

1 — ABDOMINAL STRETCH

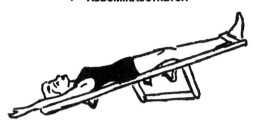

While lying flat on your back, stretch your abdomen by putting arms above head. Then raise and lower them to sides. This stretches the abdominal muscles by pulling them up toward shoulders. Do this exercise 10 to 15 times.

2 — UPLIFTING ORGANS

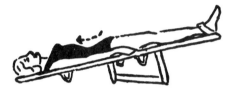

In this position, bring abdominal organs toward shoulders, while holding your breath. Move the organs back and forth by drawing them upwards, then relax, letting them go back to former position. Do this exercise 10 to 15 times.

3 — COLON REJUVENATOR

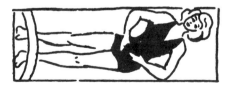

Lean to left side and stretch. Pat stretched side of abdomen vigorously with open hand. Change sides — lean to right, stretch and pat vigorously 15 to 25 times each side. Reverse sides 3 or 4 times.

4 — ENFORCING CIRCULATION

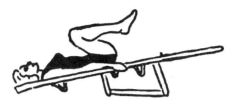

Assume this position by bending knees and legs at hips. Let yourself relax: (a) Turn your head from side to side 5 or 6 times. (b) Lift the head slightly and rotate in circles 3 or 4 times. Reverse. Repeat each set 2 or 3 times.

5 — LIGAMENT STRETCH

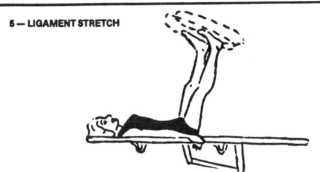

With arms at side, lift legs to vertical position and rotate outward in circles 8 to 10 times. Then change direction to inward circles. You can increase this exercise gradually, over a week or ten days to 25 times.

6 — MUSCLE TONER

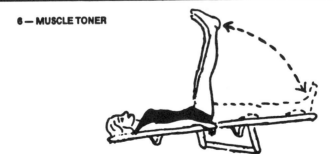

Raise both legs to vertical position, then alternately, lower first right, then left down to board, slowly, keeping knees straight 15 to 25 times. Raise both legs and lower both together slowly, three or four times. Double these after a week or ten days.

7 — ALL-IN-ONE EXERCISER

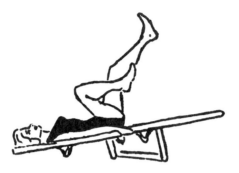

Raise legs to vertical position, then bicycle legs in air 15 to 25 times. Do this reasonably slow at first, increasing tempo gradually through first weeks of regular exercises.

8 — THE BASIC POSITION

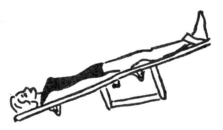

Lie flat on your back with feet under straps, allowing gravity to help put abdominal organs into their proper position. Relax completely, letting the blood circulate to the head. Keep this position 5 to 15 minutes. Note: This basic position should climax all series of exercises.

Skin Brushing [Dry]

The elimination organs are always to be considered first in developing a Healing Crisis and to work with the Reversal Process of regenerating the body, therefore, Skin Brushing is most important to get the skin to eliminate properly. I believe Skin Brushing is one of the finest of all baths. No soap can wash the skin as clean as the new skin you have under the old. You make new skin every 24 hours on the body. The skin will be as clean as the blood is.

Skin Brushing removes this top layer. This helps to eliminate uric acid crystals, catarrh and various other acids in the body. The skin should eliminate two pounds of waste acids daily. Keep the skin active. No one can be well wearing clothes unless they brush their skin. It is the greatest method to remove the scurf rum as found in the eye, which denotes an underactive skin, a poorly eliminating skin.

Use a dry vegetable bristle flesh massage brush with a long handle. It is not an expensive brush. **Do Not Use Nylon.** Use this brush dry, first thing in the morning when you arise before putting clothes on and before any bath. Use it in any direction all over the whole body except the face. You can use a special face brush for the face.

Lungs

Hiking, swimming, bending, twisting, helps the lungs to breathe more. Quick inhalations, slow exhalations help the lung structure.

Kidneys

For taking care of the kidneys, we use the proper liquids and diet programs as brought forth in this booklet through diet and exercise of the bowel.

One simple daily detoxification will take place by taking two or three glasses of liquids or water before breakfast every morning. This exercises the bladder and cleanses stagnant urine that has been there all night long and it develops the tone of the bladder. This is especially good when people pass the age of 50. We cleanse the bowel which is an eliminative organ. Let us also cleanse the genito-urinary tract which is also an eliminative organ.

****

This takes care of all four elimination channels mechanically. Water treatments may be used and massage, physiotherapy and many other forms of treatment to hasten the development of proper tissue tone and activity in the body. Always think, however, of developing the whole body rather than just one tissue or one organ.

CHAPTER FOUR

DETOXIFICATION

My approach is the natural way ... without drugs ... you may now have heard it referred to as the "Nature Cure".

There is a difference between the activity of drugs and the activity of a nature cure. I am not going to say that one is better than the other, but there is a life style that appeals to each of us ... as some people like Collies, some like Scotties, some like to be Baptists, some like to be Catholics. There seems to be something for everyone. I feel that there is something in each path and I feel that no matter what path you take, the end result will be for your soul growth through experiences.

While we are growing some of us choose to give up "junk" foods because we may have a thought that we have strayed from the Garden of Eden ... that perhaps we are living a life that is not conducive to making the best body for us or is not giving us all the action the body could possibly give.

Do You Know What It Is To Feel Wonderful?

I don't know if many really know how great it is to feel good ... feel wonderful ... and most of all feel healthy. I feel that health is not everything but without health everything else is nothing! Without good health you cannot spend your money well and enjoy it. Without good health, you cannot have a good marriage or bring up children with good health. You have to recognize that there is a price to be paid when you follow this path. It is not an easy one but the results are always forthcoming and usually are long lasting.

As to drugs ... we know that if we suppress all elimination processes, driving toxic material into the body or causing it to be retained, this eventually produces chronic disease. What we need to do is to reverse the disease and accumulation process. You can only do this by detoxifying the body ... giving it a rest, getting more liquids, draining off the catarrh, toxic materials and accumulations, which are found in the body, by bringing them to the "running stage". Catarrh means "I flow" in the Greek language and when you bring the catarrh to a flowing stage you are cleansing the body. Healing is cleansing and cleansing is healing.

Adding iron to the diet is a good way for eliminating drugs in the body. Iron attracts oxygen from the air. We find that iron is most necessary to draw enough oxygen out of the air to burn up these toxic materials in the body.

Iron is found in blackberries, raspberries, loganberries and all greens.

We want to move the toxic materials to the eliminative organs and withdraw drugs from the various tissues ... this could be the brain or any part of the body. Sometimes withdrawal of drugs brings on symptoms and elimination processes that are very severe. They may be almost intolerable. But in order to get well you will have to go through with it.

Many people under detoxification have cut out their coffee and they developed a coffee headache. We have to get out all of the coffee, caffine, nicotine, that has accumulated in the tissues to get well. We have to go through the coffee headaches to get well. The same applies to all of the drugs or anything else that has settled in the body.

People say that a "Nature Cure" takes a long time. Yes ... it does ... but a chronic disease takes a long time to develop too. We have to understand that the body works according to the law, and, in the reversal process, as it cleanses, we find we go back over the course that we built the condition on. This follows Herring's Law of Cure: "All cure starts from within outward and from the top down, and in reverse orders as the symptoms have appeared."

To take care of asthma in the reveral process, we always go through hay fever and the flu symptoms again ... tiredness, aching bones, fever. They all come back briefly, but if you will go through with this process, you will get a healthy, well body.

Suffering does not always come only physically ... it can come mentally and spiritually. I feel very depressed when I see a child with asthma being given an all day sucker or an ice cream cone. It is the very thing that produces the trouble! I see that it is a lack of knowledge or ignorance. When you know better, isn't it sad to see a thing like this happen. There are some people who just don't know any better. They learn in the school of hard knocks and through terrible experiences.

I am sick of being sick, and, I find that the average person who gets sick of being sick turns to the natural methods and to "Nature Cure".

Many people just want to get rid of their present symptoms, and we find as soon as they get rid of them, they go back on the same wrong living habits and then feel or believe they are happy.

When you come with me, you clean up your life! You clean up your mind, you clean up your ideals, straighten out your direction in life, and strive for a new body. All this involves healing crises and elimination processes. There are many people who come to me with a coated tongue which is a sign they are loaded to the gills, so to speak, with toxic materials. It means the liver is toxic and the bowel is not eliminating properly. The lung structure is filled with catarrh, mucus and phlegm. To eliminate this material we have to start the process of detoxification.

How long does detoxification take? I think it is best to consider doing it for two or three weeks on whatever program you want to go on, and then get to a healthy way of living. Eventually, you should come back to another detoxifying program according to the amount of weight you gained, the condition of your body, if you can stand it again and so forth.

Don't try to do the whole thing at one time! It is best to do these programs under a doctor's care.

A man came in one day complaining that he had bad breath, his vision was going bad, he was hard of hearing, and his tongue was coated as he had never seen it before. He said it had all happened in the past four or five months. I asked him about his bowel, and he said in the last four or five months the bowel hadn't moved well and elimination had practically stopped. He had to resort to enemas and to laxatives and he now wondered what was wrong. He noticed that the odor from his body had become very strong, and that his wife had started to complain about it. It was time for a detoxification program so I started him out by going through the Eleven Day Elimination Diet. This might not fit everybody. You must be wise in your selection.

You can go on carrot juice for five days, or take the Grape Diet for ten or twelve days as outlined on one of the following pages. You can go on a short fast, or you can go on a long fast with a person who is capable and has had experience in fasting. However, I do not think you should go on a long water fast by yourself. Always follow your doctor's advice.

Allergies are helped through the detoxification program. We find that all cases of catarrhal discharges are helped in an elimination diet program. This kind of program is the first thing to think about for any discharge or pain in the body. Go on as little food as possible and undertake a detoxification program.

Sometimes when we want to eliminate and detoxify, it is well to leave the environment that has caused all the trouble. It is best to be with happy people and develop a new attitude toward life ... this means ... you have to get away from mean, irritable people and start a new life for yourself. Happiness is part of a good elimination program. People need happiness, love, peace and harmony today more than anything else.

> We never stop a catarrh, phlegm or mucus discharge in the body. We recognize that in the suppression of that we are traveling on to a more chronic disease. We give the body its will to cleanse and putify itself and never stop a discharge. To stop this discharge is what we call suppression. To use a treatment, food, drug or live a life that stops the discharge is called suppressing the symptoms or disease.

These detoxifying programs are good in nearly every disease. They are indicated in practically all lung problems. Some diseases call for special carefulness, for example, tuberculosis, diabetes, epilepsy.

Convulsions can develop very fast under an elimination program and we should make sure someone is in attendance. In diabetes we find that a person could develop coma and it is well to have them under good supervision. Colitis responds well to a detoxifying program. Constipation is the first thing to take care of in detoxifying.

Care of the Bowel through Enemas

We do not detoxify the toxic material just by eliminating bowel wastes. There is more to it than that! We have to recognize that cells must be fed and that vital energy has to be built up in the body. There has to be a detoxification going on in the liver as well as in the bowel, lymph glands, lung structure, kidneys, and even through the skin.

Many people, having a fever, resort to enemas and that's all. They don't realize there are many herb teas that act as diuretics, eliminating toxic waste through the kidneys. The first thing that I would like to bring out is that detoxification takes place **normally** in the body when we have good health. However, very few people have good health. As we strive for good health and build structure and fiber strength in our body tissues, the body will eliminate better. We throw off the toxic wastes that have been absorbed into our tissues when we were tired, fatigued, overworked and became mentally weary. There are many acids we have to eliminate and detoxify. There may be mental acids which come from worry, hate and fear. There are catarrhal conditions developed in the body from poor foods or when people have taken drugs. Through an elimination program we can start what we call a withdrawal of drug deposits in the body.

When this elimination process is developed and toxic materials are ready to be thrown off by a strong body, we have . . . A Healing Crisis. That Healing Crisis is what we need for a so-called "cure".

Dr. Henry Lindlahr said, "Give me a healing crisis and I will cure any disease."

★★★★

Hippocrates, the Father of Medicine, said, "Give me a fever and I will cure any disease."

It is in these crises that we develop fevers. When we have these crises, they seem to be the same as a disease crisis. They actually manifest the same appearance. However, they are different in nature. We find that a Healing Crisis brings on more elimination through all five of the eliminating organs . . . skin, bowel, lungs, liver and kidneys . . . than it does in a disease crisis. The bowels invariably work perfectly in a Healing Crisis, but this does not happen in a disease crisis. That is why enemas are given when you are sick. However, you don't need to think about enemas in a Healing Crisis because the bowel works very well as a rule.

For a Healing Crisis the cells have to be fed and you have to develop the integrity of tissue so it can carry on its healthy processes with good function of the glands and every organ of the body.

There is one thing you should remember about the diets we are about to give you and that is that eventually you will have to get off diets. Most of them are for detoxification purposes, for elimination, for reducing, for chemically rebalancing the body. The time comes when you just have to go on with a healthy way of living.

A little thing to consider here is that elimination may go too fast for some people and they may reduce or lose weight too rapidly and become weak on the diet. We find that sometimes taking too much fruit and fruit juice on the diet will produce this condition. Remember that vegetables carry off acids and they carry off the acids much slower than fruits. Fruits stir up the acids and many times we have to be careful about taking too much fruit juice. This applies especially to citrus fruit. We find that citrus fruit is high in its life giving energies and can stir up toxic materials very quickly. If our elimination channels are not prepared to take out the stirred-up acids that the citrus stir up in the body, we find we can produce an internal congestion that many times isn't taken care of properly.

There are four starches that produce the least amount of catarrh when used in one's diet, and as part of this, I think that we have to consider giving up wheat and oatmeal. It is the gluten in these two products that I am convinced produce the heavy catarrhal conditions in the body. Wheat, by the way, puts on fat. So does oatmeal. And we find that the four starches that we should use that will not put on weight and will not produce the catarrh are rye, rice, yellow cornmeal and millet.

Remember This...
A long fast should be under the supervision of a doctor. Detoxification is like tearing down the walls of an old building. There comes a time when you have to rebuild and that results from a new eating regime afterwards. **Eventually you have to get off this diet idea and go on to a healthy way of living.** *It is good to go from the elimination diet to a healthy way of living, then after a month or so on an elimination diet, and then ... back to a healthy way of living.*

There are many people on detoxifying and eliminating programs all the time. They are on what I call a diet.

One man said he had been on the grapefruit diet and found that it helped his sinuses tremendously. Then he said, "I heard you give the carrot juice diet here." I said, "Yes, we can give you carrot juice as a diet." He said, "I would like to go three weeks on carrot juice."

So he went three weeks on carrot juice and then found out that watermelon is very high in silicon and is supposed to be very good for catarrh problems, so he went three weeks on a watermelon diet. When he was finished with that, the grape season came in and, of course, grapes are so good in catarrh problems, so he went on a three week grape diet.

You cannot build the body on a detoxifying diet, an elimination diet or through fasting. Find a way of maintaining good health through proper living and eating. Diets belong to doctors and hospitals for reducing, gaining or detoxifying. It is not a healthy way of living. Can you understand that ... ?

The best diet for everyone is a "Healthy-Way-To-Live" diet. You should learn this healthy way of living and use it at home.

The Physical Change Creates a Mental Change

A sick person is not happy but a well person is! As we eliminate this toxic material from the body, there is a mind change as well as a physical change because we relieve the mind and brain structure of toxic materials. We think more clearly and we're able to make decisions better. We're able to enjoy our surroundings and we see beauty as we have never seen beauty before.

These things cannot be expressed in a sick, toxic body. Sick people go around moping and say they don't feel good, nothing seems to be right and they are irritable. We believe that there are so-called mental conditions in a person which in reality are nothing more than a toxic condition that settled in the brain areas and interferes with the proper brain and nerve activity. We have to have perfect nerve supply to every organ in the body. This is the number one function that must take place before our body becomes well. The moment that we fill that nerve structure with good nourishment or start eliminating toxic material that has accumulated in the body, we start feeling better and the mind functions better and clearer. When the mind works better we find that all nerve activity works better.

What we invariably hear from a person who undertakes detoxification is, "I am feeling better!" The feelings are cleared up in the nervous structure. Our cell structure becomes hungry, thirsty, cold and painful at times. To clean up these conditions, we have to go through a detoxifying program to relieve cells of this debris in the body.

"The mind cannot be set apart as an entirely disassociated entity. No mind ever existed that was entirely free from the influences of bodily processes, animal impulses, savage traditions, infantile impressions, conventional reactions, and traditional knowledge."
—Anonymous

It reminds me of the story of the man who was buried in a cave. The roof of the cave had collapsed and the timbers and other materials had fallen in on top of him. He really needed help! Likewise, we need outside help in our detoxifying program. We need to remove some timbers, which in our case can be coffee and doughnuts, or, it can be toxic materials from dumplings, crackers and the soggy breakfast foods that people think are feeding them. We eventually find that this is the debris which can overcome us ... then one of these days we will wonder just what happened to us.

If your eyes are bad, maybe they are toxic. If you cannot hear, probably you have too much of the toxic materials from junk foods in your body. It is possible that every cell and every organ in your body needs rejuvenation. Each blood cell is made new every 30 days. You make new tissue from clean blood for a vital way of life. Let us also mention that as we eliminate the toxic materials from one organ in the body, every other organ will know it. This is because it is done through the blood. The blood contacts every cell in the body. Every organ in your body is fed and cleansed by the blood. So . . . we must cleanse the blood. We do this first through proper diet measures.

The liver is probably one of the first organs we should take care of. This is the organ that detoxifies and eliminates wastes more than any other organ in the body outside of the bowel. It does it naturally for us but we still need the anti-toxic foods. Just add some of these foods to your everyday diet. Soon you will find that the liver will start to improve and detoxify more. Some foods you can add to help the liver are cherry juice, alfalfa tablets, alfalfa tea, alfalfa greens, and chlorophyll which is one of the greatest cleansers we have. We find that Dwarf Nettle broth, peppermint, and all bitter greens help the liver. Dandelion greens and dandelion tea are also great cleansers for the liver. This is only to name a few. Then we need to have antiseptic foods and some of them are the white or green grapes, lemons, onions and garlic. In addition, pineapple juice, mulberries, prickly pears and Oat Straw broth are great catarrhal eliminators. We also find that silicon foods and foods high in sodium are very antiseptic and acid reducing.

The most beneficial foods for eliminating catarrh and for developing a greater health response of the tissues in throwing off toxic material are to be found in our iodine foods. Kelp, egg yolk and goat milk are non-toxic to the body. We find that raw goat milk is one of the foods highest in flourine, which is especially good in eliminating lung troubles and lung catarrh. Flourine is the anti-resistant element and is so necessary for us to have in fighting off viruses and infections. Chlorine, necessary for eliminating pus and catarrhal conditions in the body, is found the highest in celery and in vegetable juices. We find that silicon is very necessary for pleural catarrh (the pleura is the sack around the lung structure). Silicon is stored in the human skin and keeps this elimination organ active. Sodium foods are necessary for pus troubles also.

The best sodium foods are goat whey, whey of any kind, okra and celery. These are all very high in sodium, as are sun-ripened fruits and sweet fruits. When we want to get rid of catarrh, we use poultices and packs. Comfrey packs on sores are wonderful. We find that Aloe Vera can be used as a pack. Also, onion poultices on the neck, chest and thyroid gland are wonderful for ridding the body of catarrhal conditions that might settle there. I find that even strong sunlight is very helpful in diminishing catarrhal conditions. Altitude, dry air and non-catarrhal foods must also be considered. Bone set or Comfrey tea is especially good in relieving flu conditions and flu catarrh.

To relieve the cell structure of the debris that we have accumulated over a period of years through devitalized foods and heavy catarrh-forming foods such as refined flours, white sugar products and so forth, we have to start an elimination program through the elimination organs.

The first and most important thing to do is to take care of the toxic material in the bowel. We must have bulk and we can get this from vegetable salads. Many people don't use salads. Many people think that parsley is meant to be used just to decorate a plate. It was made to eat! Very few people take enough of the beet greens. Spinach could be used raw. When we want to eliminate toxic materials in the body, the more raw food we eat, the better is a detoxifying program. I don't mean that you have to continue going on all raw foods, but raw vegetable juices are good especially for the bowel and the liver.

Raw shredded beet is one of the best eliminators we have and it stimulates the flow of bile from the liver and gall bladder into the intestinal tract. Greatest of all ... Alfalfa Tablets.

Many times we use a pancreatic substance along with the diet to help our foods digest and we could also use an herbal digestant. We use a couple of these each meal.

There is much material built into our bodies that has to go back into the body and be redigested bringing it back into the blood.

This can be done by adding pancreatic substance to each meal. Sometimes Papaya Tablets are also very good, however, they are not too strong. We find that ginger can also be used. In addition, Mint Tea is a wonderful gas-propellant and Red Clover tea is a wonderful digestant.

The heart shares in our joys and sorrows. It expands and contracts with our moods, it weeps with us, grieves with us, moans with us, and it can injure itself in our joys. It may quiver from the impact of a brain storm whose vortex uproots the most solid anchorage. We should live longer if we could spare our hearts the responsibilities of partnership in our physical, moral, mental, and emotional enterprises. When the weary and battle-scarred hearts of unpoised men go to join the countless army of those that have gone before and the numberless legion that will likewise follow, may the rewards be commensurate with the sacrifice.

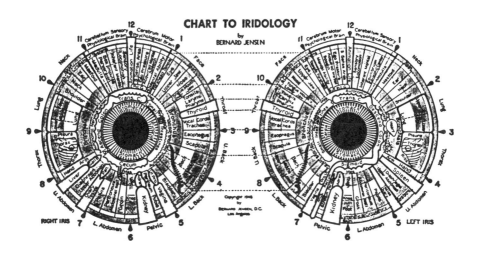

CHART TO IRIDOLOGY
by
BERNARD JENSEN

This is the chart that is used in Iridology to determine inflammation in the body, what stage it is in. It is shown in the different organ areas from a white manifestation to black. White is the acute stage, light gray the sub-acute, dark gray chronic, black is destroyed tissue. Iridology tells the integrity of this tissue, reflexively in the iris of the eye whether it is toxic laden, chemically short, whether it is under-active or over-active. The acute is the over-active, dark gray-black is under-active.

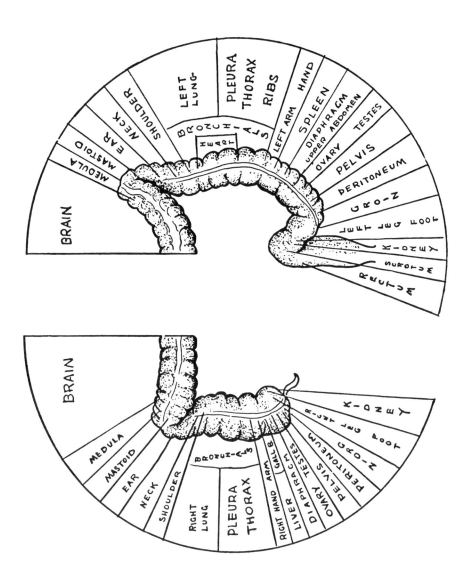

The colon produces reflex conditions in various organs in the body. The organs opposite the particular part of bowel, in the above chart, shows what part of the body is affected by the colon directly. Symptoms in various parts of the body are relieved and many times eliminated when the intestinal flora has been changed. No matter what conditions we have in the body, it is affected by the bowel whether it is good or bad. (From *"Science & Practice of Iridology"* by Dr. Bernard Jensen, D.C.)

CHAPTER FIVE

THE REVERSAL PROCESS
and THE HEALING CRISIS

"A healing crisis is an acute reaction resulting from the ascendancy of Nature's healing forces over disease conditions. Its tendency is toward recovery, and it is, therefore, in conformity with Nature's constructive principle." (from a catechism of Naturopathy)

I would like to discuss what happens after we are well into an elimination and detoxifying program. The following is a chapter from my textbook *The Science and Practice of Iridology.*

A healing crisis is the result of an industrious effort by every organ in the body to eliminate waste products and set the stage for regeneration. It conforms with Hering's Law of Cure as shown in the following illustration.

Through this constructive progress toward health, old tissues are replaced with new. A disease crisis, on the other hand, is a natural but unfavorable one . . . every organ in the body works against it, rather than with it as in the Healing Crisis. Anything that happens favorable or unfavorable . . . is controlled by natural law.
An illustration is here presented outlining:

4 STAGES OF INFLAMATION
AS SEEN IN THE IRIS

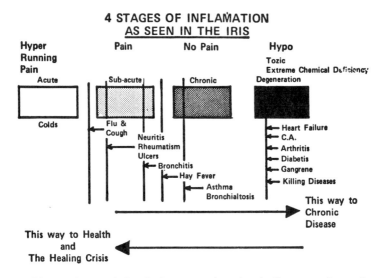

This way to Health
and
The Healing Crisis

Disease crises are devloped when we produce chronic disease or going to the right.

Healing crises are developed when traveling to the left, away from Chronicity and toward the acute stage of manifestation.

We build Chronicity through suppression — bad habits — junk food, suppressive drugs — chemical shortages — enervation, poor circulation and lack of the proper nerve motivation.

85% of diseases treated are Chronic.

HERING'S LAW OF CURE
that we follow in getting well

1. Cure from within out.
2. From Head down.
3. And in reverse order as disease has developed.

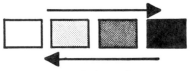

CRISES ARE FOUND IN HYPERACTIVE TISSUE
and is the will of that tissue to cleanse and purify or to throw off toxic material in the body.

Health is earned, learned.
You get well when you're
Supposed to.

The signs of the healing crisis in the iris are the reflection of an acute eliminative process taking place in all the organs of the body. Many have already learned about the appearance of disease signs in the iris. The one way to tell whether the crisis is a healing one or a disease one is that in a disease crisis only part of the body shows marked changes and the white lines in the iris are confined mainly to one or two organ areas. The reason for this is that the strong organs, which are working against the disease, will not show crisis signs in the iris. Disease does not have the support of the whole body. In a healing crisis there is usually a fever or catarrhal elimination; and every organ area in the iris will have healing signs in it since every organ is working for the health of the entire body.

The experience of going through a healing crisis will seem very much like having disease because of re-experiencing disease symptoms; but there is a very important distinction — elimination. In the healing crisis, the elimination is perfect. The bowel movement is natural. All eliminative organs are doing their part. Right up to the time of the crisis all elimination is regular. But in the diseased state elimination usually stops or is unsatisfactory, which adds to the trouble. In the healing crisis the eliminative processes have become more acute because of the abundance of stored-up energy. Whatever catarrh and other forms of waste have been stored in the body are now in a dissolved, free-flowing state, and a cleansing, purifying process is under way.

When healing lines appear in the intestinal tract area of the iris, every organ begins to show improvement. These healing lines — or **calcium luteum** lines, as Liljequist describes them — may be likened to strong pillars used to bolster up a house which probably has been abused for some time. By putting in new timber, a stronger foundation is provided. And so it is with the body; new tissue replaces the old. This replacement is represented by the healing lines in the iris. In time, the new tissue becomes strong enough to take its place in the various activities of the body. What becomes of the old tissue? It is not absorbed immediately; nor is it eliminated from the body immediately. It is exchanged by the blood stream over a period of months in a gradual process of reabsorption. This process of building up new cellular structure has been accomplished through good blood containing needed substances and through the circulation of the blood where it is needed. The real cure has taken place when the new tissue is exchanged for the old.

The health routine outlined by the doctors may extend for varying lengths of time before the crisis is reached. In a child it may be only a seven- to fourteen-day period. In adults it occurs usually after the third month. Some cases work out in cycles of seven and therefore reach the crisis on the seventh, fourteenth, twenty-first, twenty-eighth, etc., day.

The crisis can come without warning, but generally you will know it is close at hand by the patient's telling you how wonderful he feels. The final day of the eliminative period comes as an explosion, so to speak. The vital force and energies have been turned loose. This explosion, or exchange of new tissue for old, comes only when there is power from this new tissue which has come into activity. The old has spent itself and the new, built from life-giving foods and health-building processes, has grown stronger than the old, abused tissue. Tissue that has been built from poor food and bad living habits will some day have to wrestle with the tissue created from natural foods. It is plain to see which will dominate. That is why we say a crisis is a blessing in disguise. Most persons cannot realize that they have passed through a "knothole," so to speak, with the new now asserting itself.

There are three stages through which a person must pass in getting well. They are the eliminative, the transitional and the building stages. The crisis usually occurs during the transitional period, which is the time when the new tissue has matured sufficiently to take on the functions of a more perfect body.

A healing crisis usually lasts about three days, starting with a slight pain and discomfort which may become more severe until the point of complete expulsion has been reached. Following this the pains diminish. If the energy of the patient is low, the crisis sometimes lasts for a week or more. The stronger the vitality and the greater the power of the patient, the more profoundly will he be affected by the crisis.

Although there are many paths which lead to a crisis, fasting will bring healing lines into the iris quicker than any other method. Fasting alone is not enough, however, for complete recovery from all ailments. The chemical elements that are necessary for rebuilding the body and instructions for proper living should be given by the doctor following a fast.

Through the iris, you will see how the healing signs represent a fairly normal chemical balance. A person taking calcium only, for instance, would not show the healing lines as they would appear if the right balance of sodium, silicon, iodine, and the rest of the necessary minerals were included. Healing lines appear only when healing begins, and when the blood is carrying all required elements.

Many times during a fast a crisis does not occur. If this is the case, a short time on a health-building program will be necessary before the crisis will develop. All conditions must be in its favor — climate and altitude, the right mental attitude, healthful eating habits and good elimination, etc. Think of the **whole** body getting into action and correcting conditions.

Although a crisis cannot be brought about without proper diet, or fasting, the best diet in the world is ineffectual if the patient needs corrective exercises. If there is a mental state causing a great deal of irritation or colitis in the bowel, the best colonic will not cure it — nor even the best of any other physical method. Proper diet and a good bowel condition can accomplish a great deal. yet with a heavy catarrhal condition in the body, there may be many small crises to go through before the final one is possible. Everything must be considered and given its proper place in the build-up to a healing crisis.

A lady patient I had been treating for some time was about due for her healing crisis, I thought, when one morning about two o'clock she telephoned to say she was suffering from excruciating pains in the stomach. When I arrived at her home, she was in the process of using a stomach pump. Upon questioning this patient I found she had changed her diet somewhat, but not enough to prevent the healing signs from being present in her irises. She had previously asked if she could have pumpernickel bread. Since she was seventy-five years of age I did not want to make too many drastic changes or omit bread from her diet completely, which I would have done had she been younger. I had agreed to the pumpernickle bread in her diet, therefore, assuming the intake would be moderate. Needless to say, I was surprised to learn that she had been eating a full loaf of bread with each meal — breakfast, lunch and dinner. Then I realized, of course, that her pain and distress had nothing to do with the healing crisis. The bread eating had slowed down the process.

The iris gives a wonderful check on the patient. If he has been following instructions the evidence will be there. The type of healing crisis we have been discussing, however, is only for certain persons — those who desire to live in accordance with natural laws related to it.

Years ago I put a man, almost blind and with heart trouble, on a regular health routine of diet, exercise and rest. About three months after starting treatment, I was called to his home. This man was having a heart crisis. His heart was beating so forcibly that his bed was moving on its casters. I knew this was a crisis and that he would come through all right. His crisis lasted twelve hours. Almost immediately afterward he was able to read the newspaper for the first time in years. Later he was able to read fine print, and in about two months he attended a motion picture show. His heart condition was not entirely corrected but the crisis brought him to the stage of eliminating the toxic material from his body, and the building process which followed restored him to fairly good health.

Remember that when the healing crisis is in progress there is under way an acute stage of what previously occurred during the course of a disease process. While eliminating the trouble there is a step-by-step retracing. **"All cure starts from within out and from the head down and in reverse order as the symptoms have appeared,"** as Hering states in his *Law of Cure*. In order to get well, the patient must go through the crisis. You must expect it, look for it, and work toward it.

A lady patient I had at one time had spent three years traveling to various doctors and sanitariums throughout the country in an effort to obtain the healing of fourteen leg ulcers. These healed in three weeks' time due to her cooperation in taking nothing but a broth made from the tops of vegetables. No crisis occurred during this three-week period, but after about three months under my care, this patient lost her sight for two days. At first she could not understand why this should happen and then she remembered an incident a number of years before when, as a piano teacher, she had worked so intensely in preparing for a recital that she lost her sight for two days. After this lapse of time her sight was restored to the state when the disorder began.

Usually people forget what diseases or injuries they may have had in the past, but during the crisis they are almost always reminded of what they had forgotten. The eye never "forgets", as all injuries are registered there.

This same patient I just mentioned had an extreme curvature of the spine. As her healing progressed, she developed a severe "cold" which lasted 15 or 20 days. It was necessary to assist her eliminative process with frequent eliminative treatments. During one of these treatments, she underwent the retracing of an experience she had gone through in an accident 15 years previously. For a few moments, she seemed to go all to pieces. Her tongue swelled and she could hardly talk. For 15 minutes or so her body shook all over and she seemed to be in a critical condition. But after this experience was over, the spinal tension disappeared, the curvature was decreased, and there was constant improvement in the spine throughout the following year. She felt better than she had in many years.

These case histories are presented because we want to verify the rule that there is a step-by-step retracing, in the reverse order, of the disease conditions experienced through life. The retracing process is justified when we stop to think that a person's living habits and the food he eats determines the kind of tissue he has. In order to rid the body of the tissue built from injurious living habits—tissue that holds disease symptoms lying latent in chronic tissue — the retracing process, the healing crisis, is necessary. "We suffer the sins of our flesh." We suffer these during the processes of the healing crisis, which is the absolute purification process.

We should not force a tissue into an acute condition unless the whole body is ready for it. The eliminative processes of the kidneys will be more active and the results more permanent if the other eliminative organs are functioning adequately. The stomach can better overcome its problem if the bowel is working normally. If there is a bronchial discharge and elimination, the bowels will aid in this, the elimination becoming more complete as the patient goes through the crisis. In producing a crisis, as much help as possible is needed from every organ. This is why a healing crisis is more successful when the doctor has been treating the "organism-as-a-whole-in-the-environment" rather than only certain organs, as is so often done in ordinary office practice. The doctor who understands the healing crisis knows that it progresses most satisfactorily when a complete right-living program has been followed.

We can almost always predict the approach of a crisis through iridology. We know that when healing signs develop in the iris the organs under observation now have not only improved circulation, but are suppleid with a superabundance of clean, healthy blood. It is this surplus blood in the area that is going to build better tissue. Under high power magnification you can see small white lines appearing in a deep hole, finally building up to the surface. When these lines come to the surface and become very white, the crisis point has been reached. An inherently weak hole in the iris can be compared to a hole in a sock. When darning this hole, you start with a coarse weave of cross fibers, and finally fill in with a finer weave. Healing signs do not follow the fibers of the eye; they can go crosswise, sideways, or in any direction.

Since healing signs are dependent upon the degree of chronicity, the patient's living habits, and tissue response to these habits, a doctor cannot predict from the iris the exact time when a patient's crisis will occur. Keeping in mind the conditions just mentioned, doctors should judge when they would expect crisis signs to appear, and then tell the patient that they think within a certain number of weeks he/she may expect his/her crisis if that person continues to follow the health-building program outlined.

You can help to bring forth a reaction in any organ of the body through stimulation, and there are many methods for this purpose. An organ whose processes have been thus speeded up will absorb more nourishment, etc., but such stimulation to individual organs does not produce lasting effects. The reason for this is that there isn't healthy support from the other organs of the body. This is one reason why we do not believe in specialized treatment of any one organ when the condition requiring correction is constitutional. In a complete healing crisis for the good of the whole body, every organ manifests changes for the better. In this way whatever change has come about will remain because the whole structure has been strengthened enough to maintain the revitalized condition.

I am reminded of the case of a man with stomach trouble. After treating him for some time the stomach condition was cleared up, but during the crisis he developed a very severe backache. When I questioned him he could not recall having had any backache in the past, but after he completed the crisis he came in to see me. He reported that he remembered a fall from a porch when a child, following which he had the same kind of back pain that he experienced during the crisis.

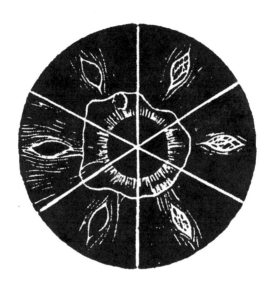

Composite study of specific conditions showing 6 stages of
healing from black and reverse as it is come in through
dark gray and finally back to the white stage.

Another patient, who came from Fresno, California, was suffering
from ulcers of the stomach. From the iris I found that this young man
had sulphur deposits in his system and, although he said he had never
taken sulphur into his body, it was there. Upon further questioning I
learned that he had worked in a fruit drying or packing plant where
sulphur was used. He had breathed the sulphur into his system. There
are many ways of taking things into our systems as we see from the
example of this young man who took in sulphur by inhaling it.

At the time of the healing crisis, this patient broke out with a skin
rash. We must always expect some kind of skin rash or eruption when
there is sulphur in the system. In an experiment once tried in an
eastern university, a number of boys were each given one-fourth
teaspoon of sulphur. Within thirty days they all broke out with boils.

There is not only the physical healing crisis, but the mental crisis as
well. As an example, in one of my cases the physical improvement

which resulted from fasting, etc., enabled a tissue response in the brain area. I noticed a change in the sex life area, where healing lines were developing rapidly. I asked the patient whether there was something bothering her sexually or mentally and would she like to talk things over with me, but she replied that there was nothing on her mind. Two or three days later she asked to talk to me and went into a prolonged crying spell. She unravelled quite a story, telling me she had lost a child because the doctor who delivered the baby was under the influence of liquor at the time. The baby was born dead and the doctor said it was because she had contracted a disease from her husband, which I later showed her was not true, but probably was stated by the doctor to cover his own indignity. This information had tormented her for many years, and as a result she had developed a complex toward her husband and toward the sexual act which finally reached tremendous proportions in her mental make-up. In my talk with her I cleared up the problem by suggesting that she had a false conception of what had happened, and by pointing out that even if she had the disease, the fast would overcome it through the healing crisis. I pointed out that there are

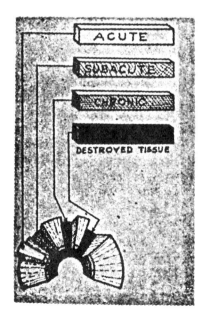

These reflex inflammations are told in the iris of the eye whether the fibers are active and white or whether the tissues have been imbedded in the pigment layer and become dark and black as illustrated above.

others who have had still-born babies and have not developed mental complexes, and that it was to her advantage to clear up this mental situation. After our talk she seemed like a new person mentally. Eventually she passed through her mental crisis, and after she returned home it was gratifying to receive a letter telling me how happy she was and how her married life had been practically made over because she now believed in her husband's innocence.

To have mental fixations and complexes cleared out of the mind is just as important as cleaning out the bowel or any organ structure of the body. In the process of trying to heal people through fasting, you will find that in many cases a long fast results in a psychic crisis. These psychic crises are very difficult to handle, and it takes considerable patience and understanding to carry the patient through. At the time the patient is in a mental state of reviewing the past. He will respond only to one in whom he has confidence and faith, and the person who is taking care of him must have a harmonious association with him. He will divulge many things from his subconscious mind which he will deny after the crisis is over. We know there are many memories and complexes buried in the mind that can be the cause of serious difficulties. I have heard patients undergoing crisis relate incidents that happened twenty or thirty years previously. Some of them bring up experiences in their sexual past which they would not reveal under other circumstances. This is one of the best housecleaning processes that could ever come to a patient. However, I do not advice prolonging a fast for the purpose of developing a psychic crisis.

On occasion I have used the assistance of a surgeon in a crisis. One such case was that of a male patient who had an inherent weakness in the right groin with lymphatic involvement. Catarrhal congestion was present throughout the body. As the result of treatment the catarrhal settlement was being eliminated through the glands in the groin. A swelling the size of a grapefruit formed. It seemed foolish to allow this mass to be absorbed and carried through the body for ultimate elimination, possibly through the lungs, kidneys, and bowels. Without an anesthetic, it was lanced and a quart and a half of pus was drained out.

Since the patient's body had brought on the crisis I believe it would have handled this eliminative process, but considering that the groin is not a vital organ, we decided in favor of draining the toxic material out through the skin. If a vital organ such as the bowel or the kidney had been involved, we would have left it to be eliminated through the natural channels. The surgeon working with me was an osteopathic physician who knew what a crisis was and understood what I wished to accomplish. The patient's psoriasis cleared up after this crisis.

No two cases are alike. Because everyone lives his life unlike his neighbor's, has a dissimilar occupation, an environment he may be subconsciously fighting, an attitude of tension and pressure; there may be 50 different causes starting 50 different diseases.

During the time of crisis there is absence of appetite. One should follow the body's natural cravings. At this time the body needs water to help carry off the toxins that have reached the elimination point and this is a time for rest. "Rest it out," is an expression I use during the crisis period, and I mean mental as well as physical rest.

The patient should be advised not to overeat during a crisis and to eat foods which will assist the eliminative process. During the height of the crisis the patient should abstain from eating for the most part, to give the body a chance to work on the healing processes, or eat only a very small quantity of food. Consider the body as being like a bank. If there has been a consistent deposit in the bank during the building process, there will be enough strength to draw upon when needed. If the patient is on a fast at the time the crisis comes, the doctor might have him continue to the next period of seven days before breaking the fast. If he is feeling fine, however, and everything seems to be favorable, the fast may then be broken.

The crisis is not the accomplishment of the doctor, nor that of the patient, directly. The body processes accomplish it. The intelligence within the patient's body knows more about tissue structure repair and regeneration than any doctor could possibly know, regardless of the system of healing in which he believes.

The crisis time usually is the time when the doctor does the least for the patient. The effort is wholly that expended by the body to normalize itself, and in most cases it should be left alone to do this job. The doctor should be alert for fears that may develop, however, and should avoid treatments which either suppress or stimulate. The body that is capable of producing this healing is making a normal readjustment and needs no outside help. In most of these cases, it is not what doctors do for the patient but what they do not do that is important.

There does not seem to be the incentive to prevent disease that there should be today, nor do we have adequate education or the health ideals each individual should strive for, to carry out his own health program. It is regrettable that some persons are merely interested in getting by and seem unaware that they are committing slow suicide every waking moment. They are not interested in health until they lose it, or until their work is hampered; then they start looking for something to remedy their condition. When such a patient has been given up by his doctors, he at last awakens to the seriousness of his problem and is frightened enough to do something about it. The nature cure doctor often gets this patient when his hope is almost gone.

It is up to the doctors to bring their patients through the crises for a cure, but they should not always promise a cure because there is no such thing as an absolute cure for everyone. It is for the doctor to decide with the patient just how a condition should be cared for, and the doctor should tell the patient exactly the way he works so he will know what to expect.

Do you see now what I mean by the healing crisis? Relatively little is generally known about it, or written about it, so far. Few doctors know very much about it. I feel fortunate that I have been able to observe all that I have concerning the healing crisis, and I have done my best to analyze and catalogue this information. The body could manifest no greater proof of its ability to be self-adjusting, self-regenerating, and self-healing than it does through the retracing of disease and the production of a healing crisis.

IMPORTANT CRISIS NOTE

A crisis comes usually after you feel your best. It is the will of nature. No doctor, no patient, no food, can bring a crisis on. It comes when your body is ready. It does it in its own time. It goes through slow or fast according to the patient's constitution, nervous system and what you have earned so that it will come on. You **earn** this crisis through hard work. It comes through a sacrifice, giving up bad habits, taking a new path, cleaning up the act that you've been in when your life wasn't working with the laws of nature. A crisis can come harsh, small, violently, softly, according to what is possible for the body to control and take care of. Some crises come in backaches, skin rashes, teeth can become on edge, a diarrhea can develop, joint pains can come. I have seen people have all of these symptoms, however, they do not usually come at the same moment but move from one part of the body to another or wherever the body is placing its energy for cleansing, rejuvenation and getting rid of the old tissue and acids that probably have accumulated over a period of years.

CHAPTER SIX

FURTHER REMARKS ON THE HEALING CRISIS and RIGHT LIVING THAT BRINGS IT ABOUT.

THE GREAT AND HUMBLE

Men who are not
bound by precedent
dominated by an institution
blinded by faith
flattered by success
spoiled by eminence
nor dazzled by their own importance—
these are the men to follow; they carry
progress with them.

Someone once asked me that when one has a Healing Crisis, how does he know if it is a crisis or if it is the disease manifesting itself.

A Healing Crisis comes to those who do the right thing. When you start doing the right thing, you can't get sick. You only get sick when you do the wrong thing and there are some people who can't reverse their particular trouble. They have gone past the point of no return.

You find that when you start doing the right thing, you do it by getting clean foods . . . you clean up both the body and the mind. You come clean, as the young folks say today. When you're doing that, you are building the good that is within you. And when I say this . . . I mean your state of health. Thus the tissue integrity develops more power, it has more repair ability, and it can regenerate better and faster. Whenever you have a better body and can throw off toxic materials, you are cleansing. You are doing a good job for yourself. So when you are doing this you don't get sick; instead, you start retracing and going back over your old troubles. For when you go back over these old problems, you start a cleansing process. And cleansing is healing.

Now, many people become disturbed when going over the crisis and when having these disturbances come up in the body. They look like a crisis and they act like a crisis. But at that particular time, we find that you are not going to have the crisis unless you have the body to go through with it. So you have to build up the body beforehand in order to get the good that can result from a crisis.

In building this body, you do it through good foods and by adding good supplements. You also do it by changing your mental attitude. We find many people don't realize that the nervous system must be built up so that the body can work better. We find the stomach can digest better when you have a good nervous system and a good mind. This is a job that takes physical, mental and spiritual coordination. You have to put all things together, for nothing ever works by itself. A single doughnut actually doesn't produce a disease. But many doughnuts eaten over many year, as well as a glass of this and a dish of that, can add up to disease.

The same thing happens in a healing crisis. When we reverse this process and start a healing business . . . well, it is like a lady who said to me one day, "I had a salad last week and it didn't do me any good." Now . . . one salad isn't going to do **anybody** any good. For that matter, one cup of coffee isn't going to hurt anybody, either . . . however, I don't believe in it. I think it is what you do six days a week that counts, not what you do on the other one day.

You find you will start a reversal process by building good health and by adding one hundred things better to your life than you were doing before. How do you get disease? You get it by doing one hundred things each day that create a disease.

Disease is really just a lack of health. Every diseased person has got **some** health. They have to start with whatever health they have and build it back up again so it is tops. When we look at a person and see how healthy he or she is, we should want to be like that person. But it took time to get to that point. You don't get that on a silver platter. You have to work for good health. You build it into existence ... you eat, drink and think it into existence. All of these things are a matter of time and of building. If you keep working with it, you attract all the good things to yourself, including better bowel movements and better breathing.

A person who isn't thinking properly doesn't carry himself or herself properly. A miser doesn't walk around a free man, no indeed! You will find, too, that a mental person who is locked up with such fixed ideas as that the world owes him a living and that nobody is any good, has a sick mind. You see, you have got to get rid of those kind of thoughts. We know that a person can be sick in the head, as well as sick in the stomach. So we have to have a complete cleaning out.

A lot of people don't realize that in order to have a good physical body, the mind must go right along with it. I have mentioned this before, that I would trust a vegetarian because usually he wants to do the right thing. He is a vegetarian first mentally, in most cases; he had to go the aesthetic way; he had to go the moral and spiritual way first in order to be a vegetarian. I don't think there is a vegetarian who follows that path just because somebody told him to do so. Something had to make that person want to become a vegetarian.

So this building, along with the healing crisis, only comes when we build a good body and good health. I don't care how low you are; if you only can wink, you can add to that and make two winks. Do you understand? You can make them really strong winks! And you can keep on going to the place where you are all winks! If you understand what I am talking about, you can have good health. On the other hand, you can only do that by adding all the good you possibly can to your efforts.

Now ... when you come to the crisis it will look and act just like a disease. So there are a few things that you will need to know. The bowel movements are usually good at this time. In a disease crisis, Grandmother and Mother used to give you an enema to clean out the bowel. The bowel is one of the first things that causes our troubles, but we find that in a healing crisis we don't have to worry about it. In a healing crisis, many times the bowels are running off and there is a diarrhea. Many times we can't understand why the bowels are so good at the healing crisis time.

The next thing about a crisis is that it usually comes the day after you feel so good. If anybody comes and tells me, "Doctor, I never felt so good in my life," I usually think about tomorrow. This is because it takes a strong body to get rid of toxic wastes and to be well . . . and now the person has the body to go through a crisis.

A well body is one that has a lot of resistance and a lot of power. I can only say this: Keep building and working for good health. Do you mean to tell me that when you breathe better air, it doesn't add to your good health? When you eat good food, it adds to your health. When you are around harmonious people and pick out good companions in your life, you find out that it is good for your health. Wise people select the people they go around with. Why go around with somebody who is going to make you feel bad all the time? There are some people who will help you to get an ulcer, if that's what you want.

You must avoid certain conditions in life and certain environments. You have to get away from a certain type of existence. For example, it is hard to get a person well who lives in Los Angeles. But I have had people get out of their car here in Escondido, take a big deep breath, and then say, "Oh, it is so nice to breathe fresh air!" Now . . . don't you think that is healthy? Don't you think that adds to their good health? Why, I know some people are going to have to stay here at least months just to get New York City out of their lungs! It is going to take a little while to do this, since they have built it into other parts of their bodies as well.

Good health comes when you make an exchange of the old for the new. The new has got to be better than the old. You can't expect it in one day, but your path determines what kind of body you have. You have got to pick out the path you are going to follow. If this path is one that includes pure air, unpolluted water and foods that are whole, natural, pure, unsprayed and not fertilized with artificial fertilizer — then you know you have chosen a good path and you're really living. You just pick out the best things in life that you possibly can. Eventually, what do you think this body is going to mold to? The greatest thing I could possibly tell you is that this body is a servant to the mind and the spirit, and only does what you tell it to do. It will follow you right along, molding to coffee and doughnuts or to a good salad, whichever you choose to eat. It will do anything you want. Always remember this! And you will find that as a servant you have to treat it well, otherwise it will not serve you at all. If you can remember that the body is a servant to the mind and the spirit, you will recognize that this body has been left in your care. It will stay here a good long time, providing you care for it properly. But it is like some of my patients — they just do anything they want, and then expect me to do the healing job for them. I don't care what you do — well, yes, I **do** care. But I can't do anything beyond what you will do for yourself. All we can do is exchange good knowledge, take the wisdom and good guidance that goes with that knowledge, and make something out of it.

Good health is earned — you work for it. Good health is learned. You will find that you have to have the knowledge to back up your efforts. I know that this is a terrible thing to say, but doctors make a living on **your** living. They make a living on sick, ignorant people. So it is time now that you awaken to the fact that you have got to learn how to live correctly. If you don't know any better, you think coffee and doughnuts are all right and that you can get by on them. But nature will come knocking at your door one day in the form of a disease and pain. When the body starts yelling, then you look to it and say, ''What is wrong with you?'' It is then that you begin to see what caused the particular trouble. And probably the greatest factors causing so many of our ills today are to be found in a lack of sunshine, polluted food and water, poor company and companionship, and work for which we are not suited. We must find our place in this world. However, I would say that about 90% of the population are misfits in society. They haven't found a good job, haven't found where they belong, haven't found what they would love to do. If you spend all day resisting and resenting the things you must do, you will end up mentally weary and with nervous exhaustion. And you'll find that a weary, exhausted body is going to be a sick one as well. Then nerve depletion is on its way.

When we talk about healing, you must understand that this is a cleansing process. It is a moment in your life when you have a crisis and the old is being left off. You don't need it any more, and you are not nourishing or attracting the former level of cell existence. Whatever you do in life, you attract in kind. Like attracts like — you attract the like thing. If you want to live on Main Street, there are people down there ready to receive you. However, it's possible you'll find out that you may have to change your address. When I say this, I mean that if **you change your foods and get away from the things you had before, the body will mold to the new things. When you come into my office** with devitalized food in this knee and degerminated wheat in that shoulder (and I can see these things reflected in the iris of the eye), then I have to wonder, how can you be clean? How can you be well? How can I get this person to a healing crisis?

Thank God, the body is forever changing and making itself over. The wonderful part about this is that you can make everything new in the body. The body works with what we call replacement therapy. You make new skin on the palm of your hand every 24 hours — not a new stomach, not a new bone structure, for it may take you a year or more to do that. By the way, I am always fair with you. I tell everybody who comes to me that no one gets really well in less than a year. You just don't blow this thing into existence in one day. You have got to get in there and really work at it. You have been storing up a little too much coffee, a little too much of the effects of a smoking habit you may have had for many years. You don't get rid of it overnight. Some of you may have been taking cortisone or other types of drugs, and have to go through the withdrawal symptoms. To draw that out of the body also isn't done overnight. But a new day, a better day is coming when people will want to do the right thing physically, mentally and spiritually. You can't do the wrong thing and expect a God of good consequence to give you everything right. It just doesn't work that way. So when you come to this healing crisis, you will find that you have deserved it.

Hering's Law of Cure deals with the activity of the body as it progresses, builds and regenerates, it uses external stimuli, the foods you eat, and internal stimuli. The end result is either good according to the health value that these stimuli represent. The same holds true in reversing the process of whatever disease we have developed and by using an evolved or a pathway that the body can develop to, or with, we find that it can reverse the process that has been developed. This is why we start from within to either get well or to get sick. It is from within that we build our good health, chemically, physically, spiritually, etc.

As we break down the old structure that we have built in the body, it develops into gases, solids and liquids that in the elimination process can be putrid, systic, acidic and extremely toxic. It can burn, irritate and produce extreme pain. This is the result of violating natural law. Dr. Hering brought out in his work that the body was subject to natural law the same as we are subject to the laws of gravity, relaxation, contraction, etc., and showed that we do start from above down to get rid of this toxic material. No illness exists without a toxic background. This is why penicillin, sulfa drugs, antihistimines were born. Normal functioning eliminates this material and so the law of reverse order goes into play getting rid of all accumulations, morbid material and deposits the body cannot use.

One little girl was telling me that she feels so good, it is just wonderful. She didn't think that she should continue on; she just felt that she ought to quit her treatments. She said, "I would like to have you check things over." I examined her eyes and I said, "You know, everything has been going beautifully. I've never seen such lovely healing signs in my life." In other words, the black holes that I had originally found in the iris of the eye were now filling in with little white healing lines. Now, when we fill them in with these white healing signs, do you know what we are doing? We are putting light in dark places. And that is what people need in order to get well: enlightenment. When you pray, pray for enlightenment. It is not a very enlightened person that lives on junk foods. Don't you feel that such a person needs more light?

In Germany, they say that black is compared to the Devil of Hell, while white is compared to the Angels of Heaven. That is why we work in this field of Iridology and put white in those black holes that you have in the iris. When they fill up with that white, they are going to express themselves properly because that is now new, clean baby tissue which comes in with power. It is going to say, "Listen — out with the old and in with the new!" This is what happens to a person doing the right thing. So we further this and try to promote a healing.

It is just like the little girl I previously mentioned. I told her, "Everything is so beautiful with these healing signs in there. You know, you are ready for a healing crisis." She said, "What do you mean by a healing crisis?" I said, "You are going to have a heavy elimination that will resemble a bad cold. It is possible that your ears will be running; you are going to have a cough and a lot of this catarrh is going to bring out the old acids and accumulations you have had in your body for some time." She said, "I want to tell you, Doctor, that I am a metaphysical student; and I have been living so right and so close to God that I just know I won't have a healing crisis of any kind." I said, "The closer you get to God, the more this crisis is going to come on. This is the cleansing time." She said, "I don't believe you." The next week she called and said, "Now I believe you. I have been doing the right thing and I have about 50 handkerchiefs out on the line. I never knew there was such a load of material in my body that had to be eliminated! I thought I was all right because I felt good." You see, the crisis comes right after you feel good. That is one thing you can depend on. So, don't go around bragging about how wonderful you feel without knowing that one of these days you are going to have that healing crisis.

A man once asked me if there are any supplements a person can take when living in a polluted city. He was getting ready to go back to New York City, and he wanted to know how to handle it. Well, there **are** supplements, and I feel one of the greatest is greens. Greens attract whatever oxygen is in the atmosphere. That is what you need. Without oxygen we do not burn up any waste in the body or prepare our foods properly. Without oxygen we don't have a temperature in the body. Oxygen and iron, which are the two frisky horses that work together, attract each other. Iron attracts oxygen out of the air. You find that New York is a polluted city and so is Los Angeles. I just lectured in Detroit and I told them that I came clean from Los Angeles. They said, "You can't come clean from Los Angeles." So it is possible that you can't come clean from any of these big cities, but I also say that it is iron which takes the oxygen out of the air.

I have mentioned this before, but it is impossible to really move and do things with an anemic body, a body that lacks the proper amount of iron. You can't even walk out here in the mountains, in the pure air, and get the oxygen you should have. You need the iron to take that oxygen in. So it is important to realize that probably one of the best ways to get it is through wheat grass juice. Just put it into a liquifier, and start squeezing out some of that nice green grass juice. Or get a liquid chlorophyll that is high in iron — or any greens that are high in iron. When you look at God's garden, you will see that nature produces more of one color than any other. What is it? It is green. When you clean off a little patch of ground and water it for 4 or 5 days, what is the first thing that comes up? Green grass. You find that animals first start on that grass. I have taken the green juice called chlorophyll from plant life and given it to a person that has had only a two million four hundred thousand blood count; and I have built that blood count up to four million four hundred thousand in only four months' time. This has been acomplished with greens, just the tops of vegetables loaded with chlorophyll that is added to the diet. This is one of the greatest things to build a good blood count, a high blood count. Sometimes this is necessary, especially so if you live in the city, because the carbon monoxide there will make you anemic. Cities will rob you of oxygen.

It is hard to get all the good foods you should have. In fact, most people in New York City have never even tasted a ripe blackberry. They are picked green and brought in to the city. Anytime you get a good blackberry, it has been country-grown. Hence city-dwellers have to get them on the outside. I am bringing this out because it is important to see that supplements are really not necessary if you live right. When you don't live right, I believe that you have to have them. So I use supplements for my patients.

A lot of people become weary in their work. Such people have financial troubles, marriage problems, all kinds of problems — yes, even people problems! We find that many times they become so tired they can't even digest their foods. It isn't always what you eat that counts, it is what you digest and assimilate. So I may have to give a digestant to persons so that they can get something out of their foods. I have seen tired people eat and never get any good out of it. It all depends on what you digest. So I give digestants to my people, and do you know why? Because all sick people are tired. Sick people can't eliminate well, and when you are tired you can't eliminate. You find that you have to develop a good strong body, and that is the idea in doing this: so you can digest well and eliminate well. That is why I even give alfalfa tablets to a person who doesn't eliminate well. Because within those tablets there is the chlorophyll, the iron, the sweetening material to keep the bowel clean, along with enough of the bulk to move things along. These alfalfa tablets get into the pockets, or diverticula, that are in the bowel and move things along nicely. That is why there are many people with bowel problems, digestive troubles and lack of iron who can greatly benefit from the use of alfalfa tablets in their diet.

There are several foods that I think you should especially consider using. If you are a nervous person and your job is one involving pressure and tension; or if you have parents who are riding you, a wife who is nagging you, a husband who is bugging you, or children who are irritating you; then you may have to have a good nerve supplement in your diet. One of the best ones, of course, is Vitamin B. And one of the greatest sources of Vitamin B is Rice Bran Syrup. Rice Bran Syrup is the food that is highest in silicon, and is made from rice polishings. Silicon from Rice Bran Syrup is for the brain and nervous system, and the syrup is highest in the Vitamin B complex. It is also highest in niacin, a natural food niacin. That will drive the blood to the head, hair, eyes, fatigue centers, ears, or down the other way to the extremeties — the legs, feet and hands. Rice Bran Syrup is a wonderful food supplement when we have any nerve depletion or nerve enervation problems.

People always want to get well in a hurry, and in most cases that is why I use supplements. For instance, I can usually get a little quicker results with food supplements than I probably could by taking the silicon from Oatstraw tea. You would have to drink many cups of Oatstraw tea to get the same silicon that you could get out of a relatively small amount of Rice Bran Syrup, to cite just one example. But in the long run it really makes no difference which you use; as long as you are improving all the time, what are you kicking about? Every day you are better and better. It is just like a certain lady from Salt Lake City — every time she comes here she says, "Doctor, I am feeling better all the time; I just know that I am going to die a well woman!" You just keep on going and eventually you get well — in spite of yourself! What more could you want?

When thinking about the common illnesses such as cold, flu and childhood diseases, one wonders if these are really necessary for cleansing the body, or do they result from improper living of some sort? Yes, they are elimination processes important to good health. The body only knows one thing, and that is always to repair and rebuild. No matter how bad the sore or how deep the gash, it still wants to heal and become healthy tissue again. Your fingernails are constantly growing; they never stop growing. A lady came in one time, and three-quarters of her fingernails were black. She said, "When will I get well?" I said, "When your fingernails are nice and pink, then you can say you are in pretty good health." It took nine months but they finally got there; they finally showed a good condition. To paraphrase a famous saying, "The body helps those who help the body!"

In the work of nature, the body is constantly trying to cleanse itself, to use every means available to make as good a body as possible. It is only through cleansing and purifying through outward measures, fresh air, pure water and natural food that the body cleanses itself.

People don't realize that we really make a cold. The cold is the beginning of every disease. Colds are common with kids because they are always in a state of active elimination. However, we have been trained to give them something whenever they are ailing, as well as to take something for ourselves under similar circumstances. Usually this is in the form of a drug that has a suppressive action and drives the catarrh back into the body, stopping the natural elimination. The drugless profession, however, says that we must eliminate — we must get clean. So what do we do? We go to bed, we rest, we go on juices, we go on a little fast. We rest, even from food. And we find that as we rest the body becomes stronger and finishes the cleaning job. We work with the natural inherent principles of the body; then one becomes the "clean man". The Good Book says "Cleanse and purify thyself, and I will exalt thee to the throne of power." Now, isn't that what you want? Of course, you want a clean body — who doesn't? That represents the highest goal attainable. And this is what God approves of: cleanliness in body, mind and spirit.

When catarrh, phlegm or mucus is suppressed and thereby driven back into the lung structure, bronchial tubes, or any weak organ in the body, we are on our way to a chronic disease. We all have weak organs. If we inherit weak organs and then suppress any disease, the accumulated material that is not allowed to come out will settle in those weak organs. This is because they don't have the power to properly get rid of this material through the elimination channels: the skin, lungs, even kidneys and bowel. The weak organs do the least amount of work in our bodies when we have abused ourselves and become run-down, over-tired, etc. So we find that after the cold the next thing we develop is bronchial troubles. When you have a bronchial problem you'll find that you will also develop a little cough along with it. And the first thing you do is to go out and get a suppressant cough medicine. The advertising industry actually tells you that it is suppression they are achieving, and that this will dry up the cough. I say that if you can cough up a cup full of mucus, catarrh or phlegm within a day's time, then you should do it. That cough is saving your life, for you are cleansing through it. But if you try to stop it, where do you suppose it is going to go? If you get over that cold or bronchial cough in one treatment, you think you have been cured in just one treatment. However, you are going to suffer from something else later on. The next day you may be able to go back to work again. Somehow you don't feel as strong as you used to, but nevertheless you still go on. You go on with the same old habits that you had before: the same pickles and ice cream habit, the same smoking habit, etc. You keep on going with that until the body can't go any more at that level of health. You are degrading your health level and you're on your way to a chronic disease.

The next suppression symptom is a little different than the other one. It is the flu. What treatment do you have now for the flu? There are antibiotics and penicillin, but these continue to cause suppression. The gastro-intestinal specialists tell us that we destroy the friendly bacteria in the bowel by taking these antibiotics. We lower our resistance, so we don't have the ability to get rid of toxic materials in the body. Now, we may be feeling pretty good again. So we go on with our bad habits of living; we don't change our way of life.

The next thing that develops is hay fever. We are coming up the ladder now; we are making a chronic disease. The idea that we catch asthma or hay fever belongs to the dark ages. We don't catch these diseases, we **make them** — we produce them within our own bodies. If you have hay fever and a running nose, you can't go to work. Nobody wants you around with a bad sinus discharge. So what do you take? People have been taught that when you are sick, have a disease or a discharge in your body, you must take something to get rid of it. But possibly we shouldn't be taking all of these suppressants. We are probably now living on knowledge that will have to be changed in the future. Also, if antihistamines for hay fever are used over a period of time you will develop something else. And what do you think the next ailment will be? It is asthma. You always develop asthma after you have had hay fever. You get hay fever after you have had the flu. You get the flu after having bronchial troubles. And you get bronchial troubles after a cold. Can you see this process that you build up in developing a chronic disease? I have people who come to my office with asthma and hay fever, and I encourage the necessary elimination through fasting, juice diet, grape diet, resting and getting away from their problems. They just give their bodies a chance to recuperate. When you build up good health so that you can have an elimination and develop a discharge, this is called the reversal process — an elimination process — a healing crisis.

Measles, whooping cough, mumps, all children's diseases are an elimination process. But it is one that shouldn't be tampered with or suppressed. I think possibly that if you got a very, very high fever you could use cool baths or a cool enema, in case there was a bowel disturbance.

When you have an inherent weakness and you suppress the elimination processes during a childhood disease, you are bound to develop a chronic disease. People bring their chronic diseases to me, and I reverse the process. Can I tell you what law I follow? It is Hering's Law of Cure. This is an old homeopathic law which says that all disease is cured from within out; from the head down; and in reverse order as you have built it up in the body. That is the way I work, because you get well when you are supposed to and when you have straightened out your life. That is why we have to find out what a good life is. Your life is either healing to you or detrimental. You have to decide if you want to go the healing way or not, because there **is** a healing path that you can take. That is why we talk about the healing process, rather than to say that there is a cure.

As I already mentioned, you will get well when you are supposed to. However, I can't tell you when that will be. If you think like my aunt you will say, "Well, he doesn't see me eat cake so it doesn't make any difference." Listen, it doesn't make any difference to **me** if you can't conduct yourself properly when I am not looking. But who is going to help you then, if you won't help yourself? It reminds me of the man who was out skiing. There is a way of making a turn on skis, although I don't know exactly how it's done. As this man was coming down the hill he thought, "Gee! There is nobody watching me here." And he turned around to see if someone was looking while he tried the dangerous turn. But there was a little voice that came out and said, "God is watching you." Just so, Nature is also watching you and watching over you. Nature takes care of you, God takes care of you. And the closer you get to God and to Nature, the nicer will be the things you can expect to come to you in life.

Now, children's diseases should be allowed to run their natural course. They are a cleansing process, but what do they develop on? Being weaned with corn syrup, inner soggies of wheat, and other things that build up chronic diseases. You build them up with bad foods and suppressive treatments. One of these days we are going to find that there are many new ways of bringing a child into this world. I think we are bringing them into the world the wrong way. A man in Europe brings children into the world in a dark room with soft, soothing background music. He doesn't bring them into the light and scare them to death. They have been in a dark womb, a dark room for a long time

— nine months, give or take a little — and to bring them into the world with light from flourescent lighting is a shock to the baby. Is it any wonder then that they cry? However, most of this Euorpean man's babies don't cry. I have pictures of these babies and they have smiles on their faces. It is really incredible! Everyone should come into this world smiling. But most people come in crying and go out the same way!

I have six children and they all had children's problems. However, it was only a matter of a couple of days and they were over it. They had elimination processes to go through, and so do I every once in a while. Your body needs to go through elimination processes to be cleansed. I don't think there is anybody living that can lead a truly perfect life. At least I haven't found very many Saints walking around! We all have our little "hang-ups", and some even have their little "hang-outs", too! The thing is this, that we don't always realize these produce our troubles. But the body is going to have to eliminate them some day. Maybe you will need to fast or even just rest more. Whatever you decide to do, the moment you start living a better life you begin an elimination process.

I believe that food is medicine and medicine is food. For example, I know that watermelon will flush out old toxic materials from the body. I know the value of a grape diet, and I know what carrot juice will do. I know what good foods will do. But you must give them a chance; you must put them in the body and let that body respond. So let up put the right thing in the body and it will mold itself to the good that is present. We are a plant, just like parsley. When you plant parsley you must make sure that the earth has iron, calcium, silicon, sodium, and all the elements necessary to make it healthy. If they are all there, that parsley will come out looking beautiful. But if the iron is left out, that leaf is going to look brown. If the boron is omitted, then the leaf will start to curl under. With no calcium in the soil it will start to wilt much earlier in life than it would otherwise. I see this same problem in people. Make sure that the body has calcium, silicon, sodium, iodine and all the other elements necessary for good health. Make sure all the elements are there for the ears, the eyes, and so on. And these elements are found best in raw natural foods. They will eventually go to every part of the body to rebuild and repair. We have a God-given force in our bodies that knows what to do with those elements and how to digest, assimilate and distribute them properly.

Nature cures, the doctor gets the fee, but nature needs an opportunity. You just give nature the opportunity to get well and it will mold into good health. Trust in God and trust in Nature. When you get a cut, do you have much to do with the healing of it? You might put a little chlorophyll salve on it to try and help it along, but that is the opportunity you give it in trying to get well.

You don't know how to create a body, you don't know how to create new tissue or how to build a new heart. All of that is automatically done for you. If it were left for you to create a body you would never know what to do. Would you put ears on the side of the head? Why are noses put on the way they are? If it were left up to you, you probably would put the nose on upside down, and the rain would run into it! You don't know how to create this body. Leave that to the Divine Chemist, the Divine Architect! He knows exactly what to do with food when you eat it. He knows exactly what to do with injections, with vaccinations, with drugs. He responds to your own "life style".

As you look at life, the biggest problem lies in trying to harmonize the personality with ones spiritual nature. We find that our personalities can get us into all kinds of problems and troubles. If you can straighten out your personality, you'll find that you won't burn out certain chemical elements in your body. You will attract something different as soon as you get your life straightened out. And the chemical elements in your body will work much better.

I bring this out for all of us to recognize that there is that mind over matter, that mind over platter. The mind is the first thing we have to think of. It is very important. Mother asked me at one time what I had learned in a Sunday School meeting. I told her that I had to love my enemies, love my friends and love my neighbors. She said, "Sit down, son, I want to tell you something. You don't need to love your enemies, friends or neighbors." I said, "Oh, Mother, that doesn't sound good." She said, "Son, you need to love for your **own** good." Her statement really made me stop and think. For I found out that when you hate, resist, or resent anybody you are killing yourself. If you don't love for your own good, you are going to make yourself sick. That is why we live in sorrow and regrets. We have got to stop that kind of living.

The best thing to do now is to get clean, free and "out with it" However, sometimes we don't always have the freedom to tell people off So you find that you have to love a person for your own good, not for the good of the other person. I have loved my enemies, and boy! you ought to see what I have gotten back. They just don't understand, so they spit back. But the higher law is this: it isn't the man who is killed that is going to do the suffering, it is the man who does the killing that is going to have to suffer. So it all starts right within each and every one of us. And this is the thing to get straightened out first.

One of the greatest things that I can tell you is this, that we live on what we pour out to others and to the world. That is why it is greater to give than to receive. There is no reason why we shouldn't love ourselves; we have to be able to love ourselves in order to love and to give of ourselves to others. So why should you go around killing yourself? You have heard people say that you are your own worst enemy. Well, why can't you be your own best friend? You should be, because you are the closest one to yurself. You should treat yourself to the best that life has to offer. I deserve the best, but I don't know about you people. If I put a poison pickle in one hand and a ripe apricot in the other, which one would you eat? I have decided which I would choose, because I know that I deserve the best. But I have decided that you deserve the best, too. So you have got to live in this little vortex, where you are only bringing back to yourself the good things in life that you are giving out. The giving has got to flow, so that the chemical structure of your body will respond happily and harmoniously. Then you are not disturbing it and are not breaking up "housekeeping". So you must learn to love people. They need it — and so do you! If you understand this you will recognize that this body is a temple of the living spirit, a temple of the living soul. My Mother put is so nicely when she said, "Don't ever try to make life happen; find out what the good life is and just let if flow through you." Then you find that every cell in your body will be bathed with light and good. And this is what most of us need.

One of these days we will find out that we have to do more healing and it is going to come from within ourselves. This is where healing begins. So I have tried to put this healing process together physically, mentally, spiritually, emotionally and chemically. In order to get well, I believe you have to go the total way. I am interested in total health. It has to be on all levels of consciousness. This is the way you get good health. What is the use in having **just** physical health? You can't do it that way. You can't expect sweet thoughts with a sour stomach. That is an impossibility! On the other hand, too, when you get married you just don't marry a man with two good bowel movements a day and a good heart beat! He must have more than that. He should also have a little love in his heart along with a high spiritual consciousness.

I guess you have heard about the man who spent $3,000 to cure his halitosis. After it was cured he found that nobody wanted him around, anyway! You must learn to live with people.

It is very important to get the body and the mind working in the right direction. When you jump with joy, you should have the mind for it and the body that is physically able to go right along with that mind. And as you go through life you will find that you can achieve this by knowing how to select things well. The wise man selects where he is going and the path he is going to follow. The wise man just doesn't pray for health, for money, or for another person — he prays for God's good to come into his life. He knows that God's will is greater than anything, and that it means good for everything and for everyone in every direction. If we have God's good, then we should also be willing to accept everything that goes along with it. You may have to go through a crisis, but go through it with good. You can go through hell or high water if you go with God. And you'll find that if you go this way you can take anything and stand anything that comes along — because nothing will happen to you but what it won't be for your highest good. So stay close to God.

My Mother used to say, "The more truth you have the more alone you will go." If you want to go this way, you'll find that you may have to separate yourself from some of your relatives and friends. I don't have the same friends anymore that I used to have. It is very difficult to have people come to my house now and expect to be served the same foods that I served 40 years ago. However, you don't need to worry about your friends: the old people will begin to leave, but you will also pick up new people along the way. And that will be good for you. That is going to be your big job: to not go back to the same place you were before. And you'll find that if you don't reach for the higher things you will never have the best of health.

A lady came into my office one time who was living in the past. I went over her condition and she said, "I don't think I will have any treatment with you." I said, "Why not?" She said, "I just remembered who you are." I said, "Well, who am I?" She said, "You used to be my paper boy." She didn't realize that I was no longer her paper boy, that I had grown and gotten out of that. To put it another way, "Annie doesn't live here any more." So you have to decide on where you are going and who you want to associate with in life. And I must tell you that you live on the last decision you make.

It is to your advantage now to take on this new way of thinking and of doing things. And when you say your prayers tonight, just pray for enlightenment. Pray for three things that will get you out of all your problems and troubles: knowledge, wisdom and good guidance. Knowledge alone will never do it for you, because you have to be wise enough to know when to use it. And when you ask for guidance, you'll find that you will have a little Angel on your shoulder who will give you the right word at the right time. If you will go in this direction you will realize that man is not made of just bread alone, of just a physical body. He is a soul, a spirit who needs upliftment as much as he needs the chemicals of the earth. As God's child, you need and deserve the best of everything good in heaven and on earth. So pray for everything that is good for you. If you ask for just one thing you will run short, and you will be leaning over in only one direction. Always remember that **balance** is the key to success is this life. And as a wise man once said, "Knowledge is so proud that it knows so much, while wisdom is so humble that it knows so little."

FOR YOUR GOOD HEALTH

Build a library of right living with Dr. Jensen's books, tapes and attractive wall charts explaining the natural way to happy, healthy living. If they are not available in your local bookstore, write for our free catalog and price list to: Dr. Bernard Jensen,

The "Man" Series by
Bernard Jensen, D.C., Ph.D.

FOOD HEALING FOR MAN, Vol. 1

A fascinating primer of nutrition and food facts for everyone, especially those getting started and working in the nutritional field. *Food Healing for Man* shows the role deficiencies play in disease and brings out the restorative power of a properly balanced regimen of whole, pure and natural foods. Chock-full of practical tips in growing, selecting, buying, drying, freezing, preparing and serving foods that prevent disease and build the best of health.

Dr. Jensen tells the story of the great pioneers in nutrition; reveals the truth about food additives, refined carbohydrates and modern food processing; shares many delightful recipes, health cocktails and menus; offers money-saving tips on food buying. Full of fascinating facts about current health-related research. **(Illustrated, Index, 448 pages.)**

THE CHEMISTRY OF MAN, Vol. 2

This volume, an in-depth study for students and professionals, presents the most neglected story of tissue replacement which can only come from good nutrition. Now, at last, a deep study of Dr. Jensen's phenomenal success in healing with foods in his sanitarium work is available. The research of V. G. Rocine, Dr. Jensen's greatest teacher, on balancing biochemical deficiencies through nutrition, is revealed along with Dr. Jensen's practical applications at his sanitariums over the past 50 years. The major chemical types of man and their temperaments are discussed in detail, along with their relation to nutrition, health and disease.

Lists of symptoms for each biochemical deficiency and for some excesses are provided. Learn how to replace needed minerals depleted by poor diets and inappropriate lifestyles. This book is a must for those who would like to have a more advanced understanding of how true healing can come from nutrition. **It should be in every library and college. (Illustrated, Index, 640 pages.)**

Charts—Beautiful color charts on Iridology, Body Systems, Nervous System, Vitamins-Minerals-Herbs.

Coming Soon!

Video Teaching Tapes—Bring Dr. Jensen's lectures right into your home, clinic or classroom with this series of VCR tapes, now in final stages of production!

The "Man" Series—The Chemistry of Man and *Food Healing for Man* will soon be joined by:

The Healing Essence of Man, Volumes I and II—The story of the finer forces of the vibratory realm and their relation to health and healing. Foods, Vital Force, Herbs, Nutrition, Iridology, Love, Sex, Children, Light, Color, Sound, Music, Radionics, Homeopathy, Kirlian Photography and much, much more! Many beautiful color illustrations.

Arise and Shine: The Spiritual and Mental Healing of Man—Spiritual and Mental Keys, essential aspects of wholistic healing. Illustrated.

Complete Your Library!
Other Books by Dr. Jensen:

Breathe Again Naturally—How to Deal with Catarrh, Bronchitis, Asthma
Nature Has A Remedy
World Keys to Health and Long Life
Survive This Day
Blending Magic
Creating A Magic Kitchen
Doctor-Patient Handbook
Joy of Living and How to Attain It
Overcoming Arthritis/Rheumatism
Vital Foods for Total Health
You Can Feel Wonderful
You Can Master Disease
Health Magic Through Chlorophyll
A New Lifestyle for Health & Happiness (My System)
Science and Practice of Iridology, Volume I
Iridology: The Science and Practice in the Healing Arts, Volume II
Iridology Simplified
What Is Iridology

Cassette Tapes by Dr. Jensen
(60-90 minutes—Inspirational)

Chemical Story	Natural Healing
Building A Better Way to Eat	Key to Inner Calm
Replacement Therapy	Breathing Exercises
Regularity Management	Pathways to Health
Divine Order	Arise and Shine
Seeds	

Now retired from active practice, Dr. Jensen offers a few Iridology seminars, Internship programs, Rejuvenation seminars and the Ultimate Tissue Cleansing classes several times each year. Write for details.

Published by
Bernard Jensen International
24360 Old Wagon Road, Escondido, CA 92027 Ph: (619) 749-2727

The charts appearing on the inside and back covers of this book are reductions of original-sized charts by Dr. Jensen. You may purchase full-sized, laminated wall charts of these and other charts, other books, video and audio tapes, as well as other educational materials, through Dr. Jensen's office.

Dr. Bernard Jensen
24360 Old Wagon Road
Escondido, CA 92027
Phone (619)749-2727 FAX (619)749-1248